THE YOUTH PRESCRIPTION

AN ANTI-AGING SOURCEBOOK

BY LAURA FLYNN GEISSEL, PHD

Copyright © 2013 by Laura Flynn Geissel, PhD
All rights reserved. This book or any portion thereof
may not be reproduced or used in any manner whatsoever
without the express written permission of the publisher, except
for the use of brief quotations in a book review.

The author/publisher may be contacted according to the following:
(w) www.LauraGeisselReads.com
(e) flynngeissel@yahoo.com

Editorial Services by Holly Monteith
(w) www.holly-editorial.com

Book cover design by Scarlett Rugers Design
(w) www.scarlettrugers.com

Formatting by Streetlight Graphics
(w) www.streetlightgraphics.com

Interior illustrations by Patrick Geissel

First Printing 2014

Paperback ISBN 978-0-9912150-1-0

The information in this book has been provided for informational purposes only and is not a substitute for a consultation with your physician or other health care provider. This information is not presented to diagnose or treat any health problem or disease.

For Deirdre and Casey,
May you always know the way to yes.

Healing is a matter of time.
But it is sometimes also a matter of opportunity.

Hippocrates
460–357 bc

TABLE OF CONTENTS

Introduction	11
Chapter 1	17
The Psychology of Youthfulness	17
The Beauty War Zone	17
Pressure from the Media	20
The Stuff We Tell Ourselves	29
Ageism	33
Chapter 2	39
Implementing Anti-aging Solutions	39
Chapter 3	43
The Science of Youthfulness	43
Anti-aging Science Breakthroughs	44
Chapter 4	55
The Master Anti-aging Supplement	55
What Is Colostrum?	56
How Science Opened Its Arms to Colostrum	60
Colostrum and Anti-aging Support	63
Colostrum Rebuilds the Immune System	64
Colostrum and Performance Enhancement	71
Colostrum and Skin Repair	74
A Healing Supplement for the Whole Body	79
In Conclusion	90
Chapter 5	91
The Master Menu	91

- Colostrum 91
- Monolaurin 96
- IgG 2000 DF 97
- Viralox® Health Spray 98
- A Word on Detox Reactions 98

Chapter 6 103
- Understanding Inflammation (and Why You Should Care) 103
- What Is Inflammation? 103
- Diet and Inflammation 106
- The Anti-inflammatory Meal Replacement Smoothie 114
- Inflammation and the Master Anti-aging Supplement 117
- In Conclusion 122

Chapter 7 125
- Neutraceuticals for Turning Back the Clock 125
- Essential Fatty Acids 126
- The Super Juices 129
- Vitamin D 142
- The Good and the Bad about Antioxidants 143

Chapter 8 163
- Are Your Feet Getting Heavier? 163
- Age-Related Heavy Metal Accumulation 166

Chapter 9 175
- Plant an Inner Garden 175
- Rebalancing the Digestive Tract 180

Chapter 10 187
- What Your Skin Needs Most 187
- The Science of Healthy Skin 187
- Turning Your Everyday Moisturizer into a Fancy Wrinkle Cream 190
- The Master Mask 191

The Probiotic Face Mask	192
The Fruit Shake Mask	196
Afterword	201
Acknowledgments	203
Works Cited	207

Introduction

EVERYONE WANTS TO KNOW ABOUT the "next new thing" in anti-aging science. Using my background as a health psychologist and health educator, I have created an educational work that teaches you a set of powerful anti-aging strategies. Why do you need a book on anti-aging strategies? Because in today's world, you have to become your own health advocate if you want to maintain your vitality. The knowledge that you will gain from this book will allow you to make the best possible decisions in maintaining wellness. The book also seeks to take complex health issues, such as inflammation or free radical damage, and present them in easy-to-understand terms with examples.

So many things in life feel out of control: your child's behavior, finding love, landing that promotion. It's easy to feel like we are adrift on harsh seas. Aging is one of those things that we wish we could influence. Another frustrating thing that we cannot control is how other people perceive us with respect to our age. Unlike for her male counterparts, a woman's attractiveness has a relatively quick expiration date based on her perceived age. How many women do you know who won't tell others their age for fear of being devalued and dismissed? This book provides a discussion on the construct of ageism and the self-talk that we adopt when confronted by idealized icons of beauty. Using my experience as a counseling psychologist, I tell you how to recognize these patterns of self-talk and break through them.

Currently our worldwide health care system is in crisis. Most doctors in practice today lack the holistic approach to the body that is needed to diagnose complex medical problems. Let's talk for a moment about medical school and why the training that your doctor gets may not prepare her to be an effective provider for many modern diseases. When future doctors attend medical school, diagnosis is one of the most critical and difficult domains to master. Beginning doctors are often overwhelmed by the diversity and number of clinical symptoms given by any one patient. To make a diagnosis, doctors are trained to isolate the critical symptoms and ignore the rest. The crux of the matter is how to define critical symptoms from subclinical, or irrelevant, ones. Young doctors are given the following teaching story: "When you hear hoofbeats, think horses, not zebras." What does this mean? The zebra is a rare animal. So when you hear hoofbeats coming your way but you can't see what the animal is, statistics say that the animal making the sound is more likely to be a horse than a zebra. Doctors are thus trained and reinforced to think of the most common diagnosis first when presented with a set of symptoms.

The problem is that the world of health is changing. People are carrying more and more layers of subclinical diseases. More and more people are struggling with conditions like heavy metal toxicity, systemic candida, leaky gut, bacterial imbalance, and diseases of inflammation. We talk about these conditions in the book along with the nontraditional therapies that your doctor can use to address them. There is also a great deal that you can do on your own with nutritional supplements and other preventive strategies to reduce the likelihood of developing one of these conditions. This book will educate you about those things that you can do on your own to slow down the decline of the body and maintain a more youthful, healthy state. Today, people are just as likely to be zebras as they are to be horses. If doctors are trained to make the most statistically predictable diagnosis, and are under extreme time pressure in clinical practice to do so, then atypical reasons for presenting symptoms will be missed. If you think you might be a zebra, then this book is for you. Holistic physicians know that there are no irrelevant symptoms; every problem reported by the patient must fit into a diagnosis of an overarching, systemic problem.

In this book, you will find that I have incorporated a good deal of information about clinical research. You may be thinking, "I'm not a doctor, why do I need to review the clinical studies on a particular treatment or supplement?" In today's world, you have to be your own health advocate. With the pressures from managed care to see more patients in an hour, doctors no longer have the time to stay up on the literature in their field. Did you know that doctors see up to thirty patients a day? That's a lot of clinical time. And after completing clinical notes and dealing with billing, your average doctor will be too exhausted to go home and read journal articles. That's where this book comes in. I have provided you with a summary of all the cutting-edge and relevant clinical research so that you can be your own health advocate when you discuss your treatment options with your doctor.

My book shares a series of breakthrough strategies that anyone can use in the battle against aging. Through my personal journey returning to wellness, I came upon most of the secret weapons I review in this book. In 2010, I was diagnosed with persistent Lyme disease. Because I believe that every dollar a person spends on her health is an investment in herself, I went to one of the top Lyme treatment clinics in the Washington, D.C., area. The physicians took a holistic approach to treatment, using natural remedies in addition to traditional antibiotic therapy, to return me to health. To support my healing process from Lyme, my physicians recommended a series of nutritional supplements to boost the functioning of my immune system and my overall wellness.

I was in a very bad place with my health. I was willing to follow any advice and make any behavior change if it could help me get better. This strategy of total commitment has been my basis for achieving success and reaching goals in life. I have always done whatever it took to make it. For example, I am the first person in my immediate family to get a college degree. In fact, I didn't stop with a college degree—I also earned a master's degree in clinical psychology and a PhD in educational psychology. I was resilient, confident, and dangerously effective in accomplishing my goals. I thought, "I know how to achieve success in other areas of life. Now it's time to apply these principles to my health." I followed my doctor's recommendation and began an integrative medical program.

Through the course of my treatment, my view of health was shifted dramatically from a symptom-based medical model to a whole-person model. I learned that illness doesn't simply just happen — we leave the door open for illness to enter through poor nutrition, environmental stress, and our behavioral choices. When I moved toward alternative medicine, I was able to find many of the answers for which I was searching. I was able to have the best of both worlds by combining strategies from traditional and alternative medical approaches. In my book, also I give you the best of both worlds: I take therapies that I discovered in alternative medicine and provide evidence-based research on their effectiveness. Using my background in the health sciences, this book reviews all of the clinical research on the best anti-aging supplements and their effects on multiple systems of the body. I give you a general breakdown of the vitamin and mineral research and share which supplements have withstood the scrutiny of science and which have not. We will talk about the controversy surrounding antioxidants and why high doses may even be bad for your health.

Most of us learn about nutritional supplements, vitamins, and antioxidants from clever marketing campaigns. Given the recent changes in how companies can advertise prescription medications, many people find out about prescription medications from commercials rather than from their doctors. If we were to buy into all of the claims that surround us, we would need a part-time job to finance our pill-popping lifestyle. How are we going to figure out which products are effective and which ones we should buy? One study out of Canada reported that supplements with good scientific backing cost about four dollars a month, whereas supplements with poor scientific backing cost up to sixty dollars a month [1]. Why are people paying sixty dollars a month to take something on which science does not agree? They do so because of the marketing plans that make these products sound life saving. We will talk about this research, and I will give you an unbiased review of the supplement industry so that you can maximize your investment in your health. You will learn which supplements could actually be lifesaving and which ones are just hype. We will also talk about evidence for alternative therapies so that you can invest your money in therapeutic choices with a high likelihood of success for your individual needs.

If you are ready to take charge of your health and feel younger, keep reading and follow the advice I am about to share with you. With this book, my goal is to instill hope and to broaden your views of how you can live a healthier and fuller life. Thanks to the strategies I experienced and have researched for this book, I happily tell people that I am forty and enjoy the look of surprise on their faces. My hope for this book is that it will be a lively and entertaining read. I have a devilish sense of humor, and I hope you enjoy it. Included are a series of cartoons that help illustrate some of the silly ways we think about ourselves and our health. My ultimate aim is for everyone to achieve higher states of health and happiness. I did it using the strategies in this book, and so can you. Finally, if you would like to connect to a community with similar interests and get great posts on new anti-aging breakthroughs, join us at www.facebook.com/LauraGeisselReads.

Chapter 1

The Psychology of Youthfulness

WHY DO WE WANT TO be ageless? When we associate youth with beauty, it's easy to become obsessed. Women have been trying to look more beautiful since Adam and Eve. Once, women only had to compare themselves to other women in their small town or region. With the global media explosion over the last century, women now have to compare themselves to icons of beauty from across the world. But what do almost all of these icons have in common despite divergent ethnicity or culture? They are all young. Men are also beginning to feel pressure from the media to look a certain way. Unfortunately, rates of eating disorders and plastic surgery (butt and abdominal implants) are on the rise for men. The purpose of this chapter is to identify and counteract the self-talk that leads us on a search for a youthful appearance. By resolving our psychic energy around the fear of looking older, we can move into a present that is focused on getting healthier.

The Beauty War Zone

How long have humans been trying to return to a more youthful state? According to legend, stories of the Fountain of Youth have appeared across the world for thousands of years. The fountain is a spring of water that will return youth to anyone who drinks from it. Tales of the fountain have been discovered in the writings of Herodotus, in the Alexander Romance (a collection

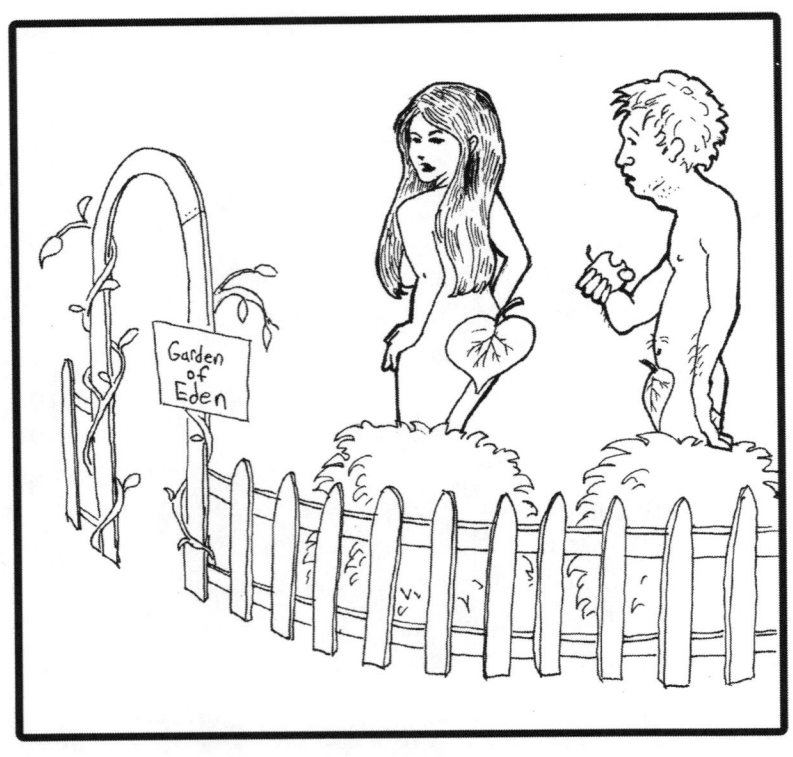

"Honey, does this fig leaf make my butt look big?"

of legends that relate to the mythical adventures of Alexander the Great), and in the mythology of indigenous peoples of the Caribbean from the sixteenth century. In fact, one of the driving factors for exploration and expansion into the Americas was the influence of Ponce de Leon, who was looking for the fountain in what is now called Florida. Perhaps the numbers of older persons retiring to Florida suggests that the search continues! The proof of this desire is the amount of money we spend each year on fancy wrinkle creams that promise youth in a jar. How do these cosmetics perform? Most of these topicals only hide the visible signs of aging while doing nothing to turn back the clock on skin.

Our culture is obsessed with youth. You are reading this book because you want to retain your vitality and discover new strategies for defeating aging. But before we jump in and I reveal a series of strategies and therapies that perform like a Fountain of Youth, let's examine our grasping desire for youth. You may think that you simply want to look younger. But I would bet my PhD that what you are really searching for is hidden under layers of unconscious motivation. Aristotle tells us that only the examined life is worth living. Have you fallen victim to our shared cultural obsession with youthfulness? In your desire to look more youthful, what are you searching for? Ask yourself the following questions:

> Am I searching for desirability?
> Am I searching for success?
> Am I searching to be the envy of my friends?
> Am I searching to be relieved of shame about looking older?
> Am I worried about dying?
> Am I afraid that becoming older will make me useless?
> Am I worried about losing my current lifestyle?

In this book, I am proposing that we should search for health, not youth. If a more youthful appearance comes with getting healthier, we'll take it. Great! But don't simply pursue the strategies in this book only for the sake of your appearance. Using the strategies in this book will help you look younger, but they will also turn back the clock on the biochemical markers of aging. As we age, biochemical changes take place in the body that can be measured. The miracle compounds revealed in this book help to return the levels of these biochemical markers to what they were years (or a decade) ago. So, if you decide to pursue the strategies I outline in the following pages, do it because you want to live a healthier, fuller life.

Authenticity is really the key to a happy life. In college, I had a philosophy teacher tell the class that as we get older, we get the face that we deserve. As a nineteen-year-old girl, I didn't really understand what he meant at the time. But now I have a better appreciation for his wisdom. Many of the wrinkles we get as we grow older are from smile lines. While at the hair salon last month, I read an article in a popular woman's magazine about looking more youthful. This article told women that smiling causes wrinkles, and so a woman should try to avoid smiling when possible. What? Stop smiling and enjoying life because you are afraid your face might age? I was shocked. But I am sure lots of women read that article and stopped smiling because of the fear they internalized. Smile lines are a good example of getting the face that you deserve. If you go through life and find joy in it, then you will smile lots. Would you rather be an older person with smile lines who found joy in every little thing? Or would you rather get to the end of your life with only a few wrinkles but filled with regret that you never allowed yourself to enjoy the one precious life you were given? Live an authentic life and tell your truth, whatever it is. If you feel joy, then let it show.

Pressure from the Media

We have all been tricked by the media into thinking that looking older is bad. As a psychologist, I really want to help you peel back the layers of mind games that have been played on you since you were little. In popular Western culture, a person's value seems to be largely a function of age. Hollywood worships youth. When was the last time you saw an older woman romantically paired with a younger man in a movie? How many times has an older man been paired with a younger woman? Like. Every. Time. How many couples do you know in which the woman is more than five years older than the man? Conversely, how many relationships do you know about in which the man is more than five years older than the woman? I would bet that you know more couples in which the man is the older party. Society just doesn't know how to make sense of it when an older woman dates a much younger man. We have to make up special words that allow us to put them in "that" group. Attractive older women are called made-up names like "cougars."

We are constantly bombarded by a blitzkrieg of youthful images. Most of our personal standards for our looks come from these media impressions. When it comes to advertising, the old adage is that sex sells. Frankly, I don't think that sex alone sells. Sex plus youth is what is being used to sell products and services in our culture. Let's examine the psychological cycle of a typical car advertisement. Imagine we are presented with a television commercial of a ruggedly handsome man driving a very expensive sports car. He is driving through the mountains, taking hairpin turns at more than one hundred miles an hour. He is cool, confident, and a master of his domain. Finally, he makes it to the top of the mountain and pulls into a five-star hotel overlooking the ocean. Enter woman. Usually ten to twenty years younger than the man, she steps into the car. He doesn't even have to pitch her a line, she just hops into the car. The scene closes with her giving him a sexy and knowing smile.

Let's break down this scenario into its psychological elements. So far, we've got man plus car equals desirable young woman. We can illustrate the terms of our psychological association with the following equation:

Man + Car = Young Desirable Woman

We have learned from this commercial that having an expensive car will get us a young, desirable woman. As it is an expensive car, we make the intuitive connection that this man is successful. Therefore, man plus car can be simplified into a more succinct term: success. Now, our equation looks like this:

Success = Young Desirable Woman

We are left with the simple conclusion that youth is a mark of desirability and success as defined in mainstream culture. Now, keep in mind that one commercial showing this relationship is not going to condition your nervous system. However, when we are confronted with this type of association fifty times a day through Internet, print, and video media, this message has a much higher likelihood of sinking in. What started out as some pictures on a TV screen now becomes our truth. Associations like this speak directly to our unconscious mind. The commercial has taught our nervous system to equate success and desirability with youth. On a subconscious level, a woman looks at the commercial and concludes that she needs to be youthful to attract and keep a desirable and successful man. If she wants to have the "good life" of fancy cars and five-star hotels, she needs to be youthful.

You might be asking, "Is it really that easy to trick my brain? Do I believe that youth is desirable simply because I watch TV or surf the Internet?" Let's talk about the power of associative learning and how your brain is programmed to learn this way. If you took Psychology 101 in college, you should remember learning about Pavlov's dogs. If you don't remember, here is the story that began the field of associative learning. Ivan Petrovich Pavlov was a Russian physiologist who conducted groundbreaking research on what came to be called classical conditioning by the field of psychology. He was studying digestive processes in dogs as an animal model for human digestion. He presented his dogs with various edible and inedible items and measured how much saliva they produced. During his experiments, he noticed serendipitously that his canine subjects would begin to salivate when the research assistant (who gave them food) would enter the room. Because the dogs salivated to a nonfood stimulus (the assistant), he concluded that mental components could control basic physiological processes. He decided that the salivation was a learned response. Ultimately, he demonstrated that by pairing the presentation of food with the sound of a bell, his dogs could be taught to salivate simply to the sound of the bell when no food was in the room. The work of Pavlov (and many subsequent psychologists over the last century) demonstrates that we learn by association. We learn that one thing equals another thing by how often we see them occur at the same time.

Imagine that we have two stimuli, Stimulus A and Stimulus B. If Stimulus A causes a response (food causes salivation) and Stimulus A is repeatedly presented along with Stimulus B (ring bell with the food), Stimulus B will begin to cause the same response as Stimulus A (dogs salivate to the bell). For a minute, let's return to our man, car, and young woman. If the stimulus of (man + car + five-star hotel) evokes the response of envy AND (man + car + five-star hotel) is paired with youth, then the stimulus of youth will begin to produce the same response of envy. The marketing gurus now have us hooked and hoodwinked. We see youth, we feel envy, we want to be desirable, and we see nothing wrong with spending down our retirement on anti-aging creams.

Let's talk about another equation with which we are confronted in our culture. This one is very simple:

$$Youth = Beauty$$

There is a billion dollar a year cosmetic industry that is able to take your money because it has convinced you that to be beautiful, you have to be youthful. How often do you hear the phrase, "She's a really beautiful young woman"? How often do you hear the phrase, "She's a really beautiful older woman"? Probably not as often. We associate beauty with youth. The best we can hope for as a middle-aged woman is to hear, "She is remarkably well preserved." Well preserved? Did I turn into a jar of pickles now that I'm forty?

I don't believe that the young corner the market on beauty. Every person has something beautiful about her appearance. If you don't know what yours is, then you just aren't looking closely enough. Perhaps the color of your eyes is striking, or perhaps it's the gentle S shape that your back makes when you lie on your side. Take a break from reading and think about what is beautiful about you. Send yourself an e-mail: "Today I am going to remember that XXXX is beautiful about me."

Now that you have thought about what is beautiful about you, I'd like for you to calculate how much money you spend in a year to look younger. Don't include things you buy to maintain your health (like a gym membership—that's about exercise, which you need to be healthy). I'm talking about those things that are simply about looking younger. Write down the products you use, how often you buy them annually, and how much they cost. Some examples could include the following:

    Anti-aging creams (retinol, etc.)
    Skin-firming creams
    Facials
    Spray tan
    Tanning booth
    Bronzer
    Light-reflecting makeup
    Skin-tightening procedures
    Chemical peels
    Microdermabrasion
    Spider vein treatment
    Laser skin resurfacing

The Youth Prescription

Hair color
Other kinds of concealer to hide aging skin
Bleaching products for age spots
Botox
Facial implants
Dermal filler treatments
Plastic surgery
What else??

How much do you spend in a year on these items? Can you think of something else that you would rather spend this money on? I'll bet you could if you tried. When we buy these items unconsciously, it's easy to lose track of how much they are actually costing us.

This year, I discovered my first age spot on my left arm. This discovery led me to have an anxiety attack about becoming old and undesirable. Why did a tiny, hardly noticeable spot cause me such anguish? Because we are surrounded by images of youthful people and are told that only youth is beautiful. Why should I endure such emotional pain over a natural process of aging? So I'm trying to envision any future age spots on my arms like the bark of a sycamore tree. When I was a child, we had two massive sycamores in our front yard, where I would wait for the bus. Because I had lots of waiting to do, I spent every day studying the differently colored patches of bark on the tree. There were light patches and dark patches. Some patches were cream colored, whereas some were light brown or orange. This coloring makes every sycamore a unique work of art—each is an original, as no two trees have the same pattern. I was mesmerized by their beauty growing up. So now I'm going to think of myself as a sycamore "in the making" with my patches of age spots. One day, perhaps I will be as beautiful as one of those trees from my childhood.

Let me give you another example of how we can get duped by media trends. Every few months, there is some new fashion trend. One month it's the high-low skirt (a skirt that is shorter in the front than in the back). Another month it's bell-bottoms.

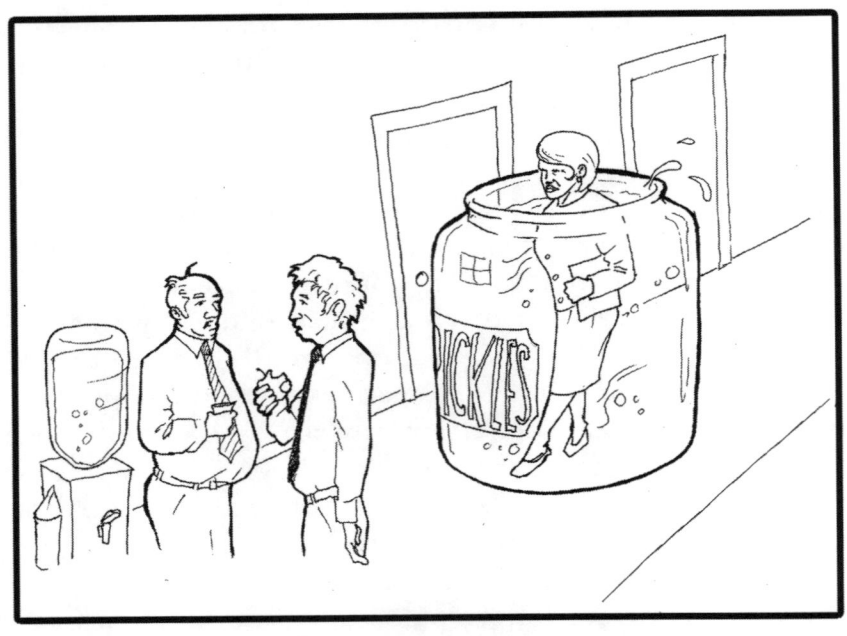

"There goes Susan. She's so remarkably well preserved."

But wait! A year has gone by, and now bell-bottoms are out. Is there anything wrong with the bell-bottom pants you just bought? No, there isn't. But the fashion industry can't make money if you keep wearing perfectly functional clothes. So we see a type of clothing for a brief time, and then (after we bought it), suddenly, this article of clothing is called out of style by the magazines. Now we don't see anyone anywhere wearing bell-bottoms. Now we are afraid of looking out of style if we wear those jeans. We have perfectly awesome bell-bottoms in the closet but won't touch them because we want to be hip.

I was born in 1973 and grew up during the 1980s. When I was a kid, there was a fashion trend about drawing in eyebrows with a special pencil called an eyebrow pencil. Caucasian women would pluck out the hairs in their eyebrows to leave a super thin line of hair; this hair would then be colored darker with a pencil. Unfortunately, a woman in my immediate family became a victim of this fashion trend. She wanted to look like all of the beautiful young women she saw photographed in the media who had their eyebrows drawn in. Over a period of a few years, she plucked out every single hair in her eyebrows; now she doesn't have any. She has an unfortunate and constant look of surprise on her face. Because she has no eyebrows, she has to draw them on every day. Also unfortunate is the fact that she sometimes draws them on badly—one will be higher than the other or one thicker than the other. She jokes, "Some people have bad hair days. I have bad eyebrow days." Now fashion trends have changed and eyebrows are back in. Because she bought into a beauty fad, she has permanently disfigured her face. Take a moment and list some of the fashion or beauty trends you have bought into over the years. How much money have you wasted on things that go out of style? My personal shopping habits are to try to stick to things that are timeless—little black dresses, pencil skirts, knitted cable textiles, pressed white shirts, silks and wool. I try to buy items that can go with everything—like red handbags and shoes that work with both black and brown palettes. You don't need the latest thing to look good.

As cultures move into industrial and technological economies, they become increasingly image conscious. It has been estimated that one national economy spent over a billion dollars a year on these products. But do the products we buy even work? Before spending your grocery money on expensive skin care products that promise the Fountain of Youth, consider this study conducted in Sweden. Everyone knows that they know about beauty in Sweden; Scandinavian women are considered to be among the most beautiful in the world. So I took note when researchers in Sweden looked at the influence of product presentation on acceptance of wrinkle creams. This study investigated whether the appearance of luxury packaging affected how women perceived the effectiveness of wrinkle creams [2]. Eighty Swedish women were assigned to one of three groups: an expensive wrinkle cream in a luxury jar, a regular moisturizer in a luxury jar, and an expensive cream in a neutral jar. The women treated their skin for six weeks and then conducted a self-evaluation. Also, a trained observer clinically evaluated their skin, while skin smoothness was measured by optical profilometry. The researchers could not verify that the luxury cream performed better than the regular moisturizer. The women and objective measurements both indicated that the two creams had the same effect on skin. Interestingly, participants who were given the luxury jar tended to use more product over the six-week trial than those given the neutral jar. So, when blinded, subjects thought that the regular moisturizer performed as well as the expensive cream. Still want to plunk down all that money at the cosmetic counter? You need to ask yourself the following questions:

- In this economy, can I really afford to be spending this much money on my appearance?
- In this economy, can I really afford to be spending this much money on products that don't do what they promise to do?

All of us want to protect ourselves from aging. But in this chapter, I am proposing that we focus on increasing our health instead of falling for fear-based strategies about aging. Now, maybe you think that you need a retinol-based product for your wrinkles (you won't once you follow my recommendations). But let's just say that you still think your skin will benefit from it. Then simply look into what drug stores offer a retinol-based product and switch to that. Remember, the Swedish study suggests that high cost is unrelated to effectiveness. You will likely be able to get the benefit for which you are looking from a much cheaper product.

The Stuff We Tell Ourselves

Despite scientific findings, we continue to purchase high-priced wrinkle creams because we think that they work better than cheaper ones. But if the Swedish study results are correct, there is no relationship between cost and effectiveness. High-priced wrinkle creams and supplements work no better than many of their lower-cost alternatives. So why are we convinced that the expensive brands work better? The answer probably lies in a psychological construct called *cognitive dissonance*. The idea of cognitive dissonance has been around since the time Aesop wrote his famous fables. In a fable called "The Fox and the Grapes," a fox tried his hardest to reach a bunch of grapes in a tree. Because he was unable to reach them, he decided that he never wanted the grapes in the first place. This story is the origin of the expression "sour grapes." When someone accuses us of "sour grapes," we are pretending not to care for something we really want *because* we can't have it. Modern social psychology has taken this very old concept and explored it in depth.

Cognitive dissonance describes the phenomenon that people are uncomfortable when they are asked to believe two things that are very different. If I want the grapes, but I cannot get to them, then I am uncomfortable. In other words, when two beliefs are very different, it causes us distress to cognitively subscribe to both. Instead of living in distress, we have the option of changing or replacing one of these beliefs. In this situation, we are highly motivated to massage our beliefs to reduce anxiety. We decide that we never wanted the grapes anyway. To illustrate cognitive dissonance, I want to discuss the beliefs our culture held with regard to seatbelts. Back before seatbelt laws were instituted, people just didn't want to be bothered to click a seatbelt every time they got into a car. It was too much work. Then evidence from accident data started coming out that seatbelts saved lives. Despite this evidence, people still didn't want to wear a seatbelt. But now they were left with two very divergent beliefs:

"I don't want to wear a seatbelt."
"Seat belts save lives."

So what happened to the group psychology of our culture? People were in distress because they believed that seatbelts saved lives, but they weren't wearing them. Then someone started circulating the belief that to survive a car accident, you needed to be thrown from the car. I have a clear memory of my mother telling me to stop wearing a seatbelt because getting thrown from the car was my best option in an accident. People were able to drop the second belief to resolve their distress. Their new beliefs looked like this:

"I don't want to wear a seatbelt."
"Not wearing a seatbelt could save my life."

With these new beliefs in place, people didn't have to feel anxiety over not wearing a seatbelt. They reduced their cognitive dissonance by changing one of their beliefs.

Fortunately, more data were released showing that most people thrown from their cars did not survive the accident.

People were put back into a state of cognitive dissonance with the first two beliefs we discussed. This time, they resolved their anxiety by buckling up.

I would like to propose that a similar thought process is going on with our beliefs about wrinkle creams and high-priced supplements. Let's examine our beliefs about wrinkle creams, just like we did with attitudes toward seatbelts. Likely, one of my beliefs is, "Only things that are expensive work well." This belief is summarized by the common saying that "you get what you pay for." Because I believe that only expensive things work, I go out and plunk down the dough for an expensive wrinkle cream. Over the next few weeks, I pay close attention to the quality of my skin. I now choose a second belief from these two options:

"This wrinkle cream worked."
"This wrinkle cream didn't work."

Take a look at the following belief pairings and guess which belief combination has the most cognitive dissonance associated with it. (This is the combination that causes the most distress and therefore is the one that people will avoid.)

<u>Combination 1</u>
"Only things that are expensive work well."
"This wrinkle cream worked."

<u>Combination 2</u>
"Only things that are expensive work well."
"This wrinkle cream didn't work."

Correct! Combination 2 causes the most cognitive dissonance and is the one that people will want to avoid. How would you feel if you spent a lot of money on a wrinkle cream and it didn't work? Your feelings might include frustration, anger, embarrassment, feeling cheated, loss, and disappointment.

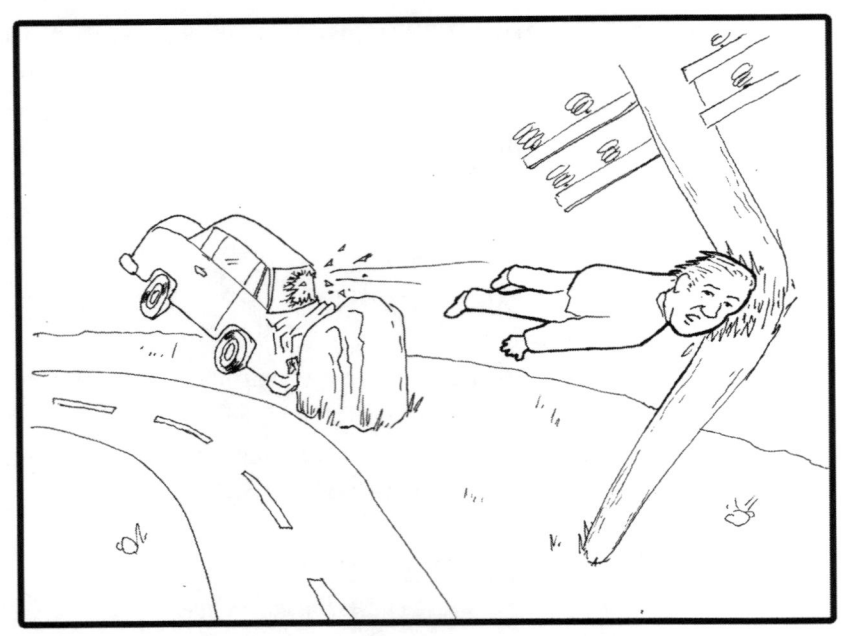

"Good thing I didn't have a seatbelt on."

These are all feelings that people want to avoid. So which belief pair do they choose? They choose the first one, in which they tell themselves that the wrinkle cream worked, *even if it didn't!* If the Swedish study is true and you just spent seventy-five dollars on a tiny canister of cream, then you are likely to convince yourself that it improved your skin, even if it didn't perform any better than the drugstore brand.

Ready to put your money on the table? If you would like to perform a similar study on yourself, I invite you to do so. Here is how you might go about it: Purchase two small, clean canisters. Put your expensive wrinkle cream in one and a similar, cheaper product in the other. (Or have someone else do it to make the identity of the creams even more secure.) Now, mix up the canisters so you don't know which is which. Use each one for six weeks at a time. Do you see a change in the quality of your skin when you switch canisters, or does your skin look the same? If you don't see a difference, then I would recommend going with the cheaper brand in the future.

Ageism

There is a term that sums up our negative feelings about getting older: *ageism.* Ageism is a negative attitude toward other people because of their age. It leads to discrimination against older persons and contributes to the fear that young people have about looking older. Ageism is apparent in many social structures across the globe, but it is the most prevalent in the West. If a social stigma exists against older persons, then I will be more likely to feel negative about my own aging process. Our culture encourages us to direct the negative feelings of ageism toward ourselves as we get older. This is called *internalized ageism.* Because I feel more negative about my own aging process, I am more likely to support the cosmetic and cosmetic dermatology industry. This fear of aging can drive us to extreme measures, including surgery or other highly expensive procedures, to reduce the signs of visible aging.

As a psychologist, I have to ask, how can we reduce internalized ageism and feel more positive about this very natural and inevitable process? Researchers from Israel at the Interdisciplinary Department of Social Sciences have offered a few strategies [3]. As we age, we need to ensure that our self-worth remains high. One way to maintain our self-worth as middle-aged and older adults is to contribute to the development of younger persons. If you work, find an opportunity to mentor a younger colleague. Share all of your wisdom and experience to help that person be more successful in his career. If you don't work, find a volunteer outreach program through which you can contribute to the growth of someone younger than you.

In all seriousness, I blame the invention of the printing press for the rise of ageism in our culture. Before we had books, we had to rely on the storytelling of older people for survival. Where were the best fishing grounds? Which plants were edible, and where did they grow? Which people were related? Having an older person answer these questions could mean the difference between life and death. Young people looked to older people to repeat these stories over and over until they were memorized for the next generation. Even if the elderly were too frail to hunt or gather, they still had an essential part to play in society. When we became able to write this knowledge down and mass-produce it for distribution, we no longer needed older people to perform as the repository of the culture's knowledge. Older people lost their place and value.

Even though we can now write down our knowledge, we need to find ways for older persons to pass on their experience to others. Many types of knowledge are more difficult to pass on in written form, for example, how to improve our soft skills such as communication and personal acumen; how we might use influence to accomplish goals within a defined organizational structure; and how to endure the trials of romantic love. Young people today still make the same mistakes in romance as people did five hundred years ago. An experienced, wise adult can add value through mentoring. Mentoring improves the self-worth of older persons and helps to defeat internalized ageism.

The Youth Prescription

Bodner [3] also recommends a few other strategies to reduce internalized ageism. At the risk of getting on my soapbox, I'd like to touch on another important point of his work. Bodner talks about weakening the effects of age stereotypes in the media. Think about all of the instances in which you have seen older people portrayed as stupid, confused, and worthy of ridicule. If we want young people to value our older adults, we have to stop depicting them in such devalued terms.

What does it mean to age gracefully? The strategies I describe in this book will help you age more gracefully. But we have to prepare middle-aged adults for living healthy lives as older adults. It is a fact that we will not be young forever. Instead of clinging desperately to their lost youth, middle-aged adults need to come to a place of acceptance of their aging. Think about the last older woman with whom you interacted who was clinging to her lost youth. Perhaps she was dressed in a skirt that was too short, covered in thick makeup, and showing face-lift scars around a receding hairline. Unnatural and desperate are always ugly. I would encourage the readers of this book to pursue the strategies I outline in the service of health and having a full life. You will get the face that you deserve.

You may have come to this book with the belief that the media does not influence how you feel about your own aging. However, social psychologists have been able to document the influence of the media in creating disorders of body image. For example, there is a *dose–response relationship* between media exposure and eating disorder symptoms. That means that more exposure to skinny models in the media leads to greater reports of eating disorder symptoms; the media does make us feel bad in comparison to an idealized icon of beauty [4]. Just as "you are what you eat" holds true for nutrition, "you are what you see" holds true for self-concept. What else defines these icons of beauty besides abnormally low body weight? They are all youthful. You just can't find work as a model once you hit your thirties. The more we are exposed to this youthful, idealized, unattainable formula for beauty, the greater the risk of mental distress and poor self-concept. Psychologists have even declared that the stigma of aging can severely impact an individual's well-being, body image, and quality of life [5]. These researchers recommend that, before any dermatological treatment, the patient be evaluated for psychological distress and distorted body image.

This media pressure doesn't just affect women; men are also vulnerable. For those of you thinking that the demonization of the media is a tired feminist narrative, know that young men are also negatively impacted by the media. Men's body dissatisfaction also increases when they are exposed to images of attractive young men [6]. We are left with the conclusion that ageism is on the rise for men as well as women.

As we move into middle age and beyond, our satisfaction with our bodies goes down. Advertising uses youth to sell products. The underlying schema of these ads is that if you buy and use our products, you will be young forever. When was the last time you saw an older woman promoting a car, cosmetic, juice drink, necklace, or nutritional supplement? The only time that you see an older person promoting a product is when that product is bought almost exclusively by the elderly. Aging is a normal physiological process, but as aging moves us further away from the ideal, we are more likely to experience body dissatisfaction [7]. These age-related body image issues can lead to food restriction, depression, social withdrawal, impaired self-worth, and disorders of eating. Our culture's glorification of youth leaves the middle-aged emotionally and financially bankrupt.

The next time you are watching TV or surfing the Internet, try defining the implicit associations in the advertisements, like we did for the car ad earlier in this chapter. Try asking the following questions, and you will begin to see through the house of cards on which most advertising is built:

- What was my first feeling when I saw this advertisement?
- What was my first thought when I saw this advertisement?

- What idealized world will I get if I make the purchase in the advertisement?

- Would I really get that idealized world by making the purchase?

- How is this advertisement using fear to get me to make the purchase?

- What nonidealized world will I be left with if I don't make the purchase?

Fortunately, the brain is plastic. This means that we can retrain the nervous system to make the associations that we consciously choose for ourselves. Instead of experiencing lower self-concept and envy when presented with images of youth, you can build different associations in your brain that you control. Instead of feeling envy, what would it be like to feel compassion for the youthful model in the media? These icons of attractiveness are so completely caught up in the delusion of their own making that they may never escape. As soon as a beauty icon gets her first wrinkle, her foundation of self-concept will come crashing down. Choosing compassion is perhaps the best road out of our own fear-based delusions about aging. It's impossible to feel fear and love at the same time. Now that you have practiced feeling compassion for the object of your former envy, let's try an even harder exercise. What would it be like to now offer that compassion to yourself? It's impossible to feel fear about your own aging process when your heart opens in compassion. Give it a try — you deserve it.

CHAPTER 2

IMPLEMENTING ANTI-AGING SOLUTIONS

IN THIS BOOK, WE DISCUSS the scientific findings on a number of nutritional supplements and health concerns. As I make no money on the supplement industry, I have tried to give you an unbiased evaluation of these therapies. Most nutritional supplements out there have very limited scientific backing. The marketing you see touting the benefits of a supplement is often based on the findings of a single study. Suddenly we are supposed to believe that this product will solve all of our health problems. After being an academic in the scientific community for many years, I can speak expertly to the fact that one study showing efficacy proves nothing. If you look hard enough, I am certain that you can find one study reporting a health benefit of arsenic—but that doesn't mean that you should start taking it. Before you start taking a supplement, it should have demonstrated efficacy across researchers, experimental methods, and time. Before you invest your money and health in something, make sure that there is general scientific agreement about its effect on your body. In this book, I discuss supplements that have gone through this very validation process.

Next, you want to make sure that you are taking the same dose that studies used to demonstrate efficacy. If scientific research shows an effect for one gram of vitamin C a day, then it doesn't do you any good to only take one hundred milligrams of it. If you want the clinical effect, then you have to take the clinical dose. Lastly, not all supplements are made the same.

Remember, the supplement industry is not a charity organization, only interested in your welfare. These are businesses that are trying to reduce costs and maximize profits. Make sure that you choose a product that is not padded out with fillers or sourced from substandard methods. What do I mean by this? If you are well versed in the supplement world, you may know that calcium can be obtained from different sources. In nature, calcium exists only in combination with other substances such as calcium carbonate, calcium citrate, and calcium phosphate. These different sources vary in expense and also in how easily they are absorbed in the body. If your supplement manufacturer has cut costs too severely, then you may be taking a product that does not have a high enough bioavailability to be effective. In some cases, the cheaper product may not be the better buy.

Talk to your doctor before taking any of the supplements reviewed in this book, especially if you have significant health problems or take medications. The material in this book is designed to provide information about supplements that have been obtained through scientific methods and research. However, this book is not designed to be a substitute for a consultation with a physician or other qualified health care provider about your medical condition. This book is not intended to diagnose, treat, or cure any disease or to prescribe any medically active substance. Rather, the contents of the book are designed to educate you so that your conversations with your physician about your medical status can be more productive.

This book summarizes a body of knowledge to be used when talking to your doctor about what interventions can be most beneficial to you based on your presenting problem and medical history. These supplements have the potential to be of great benefit, but you should not begin supplements without talking to your doctor first. A basic rule of thumb is that you should consult with a medical professional before beginning *any* new conventional or alternative therapy. Finally, these statements on dietary supplements have not been evaluated by the U.S. Food and Drug Administration (FDA). Different views on these topics may appear in other articles or publications. Other publications may also use other scientific studies to draw different conclusions about the efficacy of the therapies reviewed in this book.

Chapter 3

The Science of Youthfulness

From chapter 1, we can conclude that we are under enormous pressure to look a certain way. But there may be something to looking young that goes beyond media pressure. In fact, there may be health-conscious lifestyle factors that are correlated with a youthful appearance. There is evidence to suggest that looking younger is directly related to healthy habits. Although we may value youth because the media tells us to do so, we may also value a young-looking appearance because we associate it with health. Looking young may be related to improved physical function, enhanced cognitive function, and increased survival [8]. When women in Shanghai, China, were studied, ratings of a youthful appearance for women were correlated with greater years of education, frequency of visiting one's doctor, spending less time in the sun, and greater levels of physical activity. If someone wants to look young for her age, she has to choose healthy behaviors early.

Most of us want to look younger. But the foundation of youth is the feeling of health and vitality that we had when we were younger. No matter what your age, it's never too late to start taking care of yourself. The strategies outlined in this book will help you live a healthier life; this renewed health will shine out of you. Getting your sparkle back isn't just about looking good, it's about healing yourself from the inside out.

Laura Flynn Geissel, PhD

ANTI-AGING SCIENCE BREAKTHROUGHS

This chapter reviews some of the best anti-aging breakthroughs to come out in the last decade. These are my top trends in anti-aging science, both for their potential for human healing and in terms of new product development. Be on the lookout for these new treatments and products.

The love drug cosmetic. Your husband's Viagra may be your next secret weapon in the battle against cellulite. It may seem that no matter how much you exercise, cellulite just won't quit. Cellulite is, in essence, excess fat under the skin. The pathophysiology of the causes of cellulite are complex and poorly understood. Conventional treatments for cellulite all involve increasing microcirculation under the skin so that the excess fat is processed more efficiently. With more blood flow to the area, fat is removed at a faster rate. These treatments can include ultrasound, thermotherapy, pressotherapy, and using electrical stimulation to break up the fat. Attempts to treat cellulite with orally administered medications have not been very effective. However, researchers have shown that high doses of Viagra lead to a breakdown of lipids (fat) in cultured fat cells [9]. They proposed that topical applications of Viagra can both break down fats and increase blood circulation in the skin to help process excess fat. Viagra has the potential to increase microcirculation just like the accepted, conventional therapies for cellulite. If Viagra can get enough blood in the penis to stimulate an erection, it is likely that it can mimic the effects of other cellulite treatments that increase blood flow to the skin. Good-bye cellulite.

The wrinkle-resistant wardrobe. Researchers at the Advanced Chemical Institute of Catalonia in Barcelona, Spain, have proposed antioxidant-infused fabric called cosmetotextiles [10]. One of the latest media crazes over anti-aging supplements is over resveratrol. This naturally occurring compound is believed to act as an antioxidant, deactivating free radicals. We will talk more about this supplement later on in the book; for now, just remember that this is a natural antioxidant found in many foods. The researchers in Barcelona proposed that this compound can be used to protect the skin from free radicals and oxidative stress. But when we take or use an antioxidant, how do we really know if it is capturing free radicals and neutralizing them? The researchers in this study used a very clever methodology to independently verify the free radical neutralizing power of topically applied resveratrol. After making an alcohol solution of resveratrol and using an animal model, they applied it topically to the skin. They then separately examined each layer of the skin using DPPH radical inhibition.

When you administer a chemical called DPPH, it binds to free radicals and changes from a deep purple color to yellow in the process. If you have an effective amount of antioxidant on board, like resveratrol, you should observe less conversion of DPPH from purple to yellow because there are fewer free radicals with which it can react. Using this chemistry and an assay of the three layers of skin (stratum corneum, epidermis, and dermis), the researchers were able to determine what topical dose of resveratrol was needed to penetrate all three layers of the skin and provide free radical protection. They then used fabric infused with resveratrol to deliver the same dose to the skin. The researchers concluded that fabric infused with antioxidants can deliver highly effective free radical protection to the skin. We will talk later about the difficulty of getting enough orally administered antioxidants to the outer layers of the skin that need it. With this in mind, topical applications of antioxidants through special clothing may be in our future.

The balance balm. Hormones are the chemical messengers that the body uses to control metabolism, the sleep-wake cycle, sexuality, and other bodily functions. When hormones get out of balance, they play a big role in the aging process. As our hormones decline with age, their natural balance is disrupted,

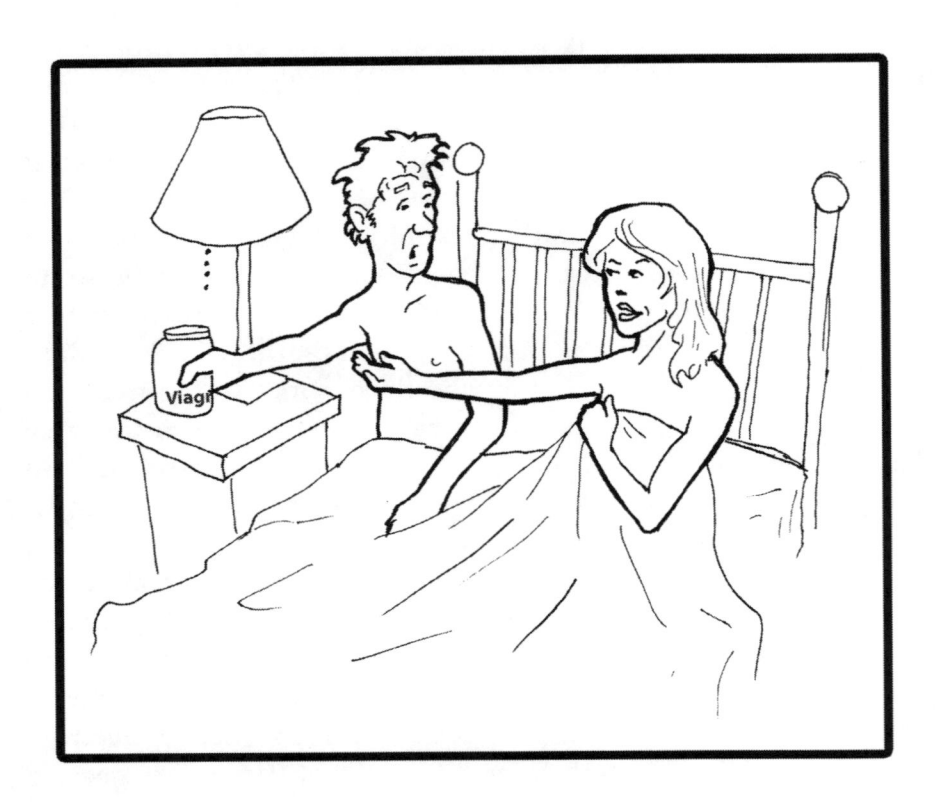

"Hand it over, honey."

and the body's repair mechanisms slow down. When repair mechanisms slow down, we start to age.

A number of studies have recently been conducted that examine the effect of topically applied growth hormone on skin as a new anti-aging strategy. If we can deliver hormones directly to the skin, these chemical messengers for cell repair can reverse aging for the skin. In one study, 83 percent of subjects using a human growth hormone cream for sixty days reported improvement in wrinkles around the eyes [11]. In another piece of work [12], patients using a human growth factor cream after a micro laser peel reported fewer side effects such as edema, crusts, and burning. Another group of subjects using a human growth factor cream with caffeine also reported significant improvement [13]. As you watch the skin care market, you will see more and more hormone-based wrinkle creams hitting shelves near you.

Not your mother's jeans. Gene therapy may be the bold new frontier for anti-aging science. The rate at which our youthful functioning declines with age is determined by certain sequences of our DNA called genes. People are born with different genes; that is why we all look a little differently from one another. One aging pathway I would like to discuss is the biochemical process of methylation, a major biochemical process for breaking down cellular waste and toxins. Methylation occurs in the body about a billion times a second in the liver during detoxification. Multiple genes are involved in making the enzymes for methylation. Unfortunately, some people are missing some, or all, of the genes responsible for making the enzymes that do the work of methylation. If one person has all the genes used in the methylation pathway but another person is missing one, then this second person may be more vulnerable to premature aging. Why? Because our second person does not process toxins the way she is supposed to. As these chemical wastes build up, they can interfere with biochemical reactions, and the person ages more quickly. Faulty methylation has been linked to a number of health problems, including cancer, cervical dysplasia, and impaired DNA repair. Impaired methylation is very common, with up to one-third of people missing DNA code for making all of the enzymes in the methylation pathway. You can be tested with a simple blood test for methylation enzymes, and your holistic physician can recommend nutritional supplements to increase your rates of methylation if you are deficient.

What if we could act directly on our DNA to prevent age-related errors and dysfunction? Researchers are starting to investigate how the biochemical markers of aging can be traced back to *which* and *how* DNA is coded into enzymes and chemical messengers. We can now evaluate topical cosmeceuticals for how they impact the genes we know to be related to aging [14]. To help establish a process for evaluating the gene modulation effect of anti-aging cosmeceutical ingredients, researchers looked at *Aframomum angustifolium* seed extract and *Malva syvestris* extract. Both of these anti-aging treatments were shown to modify the genes in the recipient cells, and both are known to improve the visible appearance of skin by reducing age-related changes. *A. angustifolium* was shown to modify antioxidant genes (*metallothionein 1*, *metallothionein 2*, *thioredoxin*, and *glutathione peroxidase*), resulting in an increase in antioxidant efficiency. Resea also found that *M. syvestris* modified the same genes that are affected by retinoic acid, a metabolite of Retin-A that stimulates skin repair. As the science of anti-aging cosmeceuticals and supplements marches forward, we should look for products with the proven ability to correct errors in our DNA expression that cause us to age prematurely. You no longer have to settle for moisturizers that only plump up the skin to hide aging; you can repair the skin at its most basic level.

You don't always get what you pay for. Most dermatologists believe that topical antioxidants will improve the health of skin. Topical antioxidants can protect the skin from photoaging, wrinkles, and inflammation and can affect intracellular signaling pathways involved in the aging of skin [15]. But how do we know for sure which products improve the health of skin? With so many topical skin care options on the market, which ones do we choose? One group of researchers has attempted to quantify the extent to which topical creams provide protection from reactive oxygen species, or free radicals. They wanted to find out which creams provide the benefits they claim in their marketing materials. Using a chemical test for free radical neutralization called the Briggs–Rauscher reaction, researchers found that many dermocosmetic products do demonstrate their claims of free radical protection. However, the protective effect was quite variable across wrinkle creams and was not correlated to price. Similar to what was found in the Swedish study discussed in chapter 1, some inexpensive creams perform better than expensive ones. It is hoped that the future of wrinkle creams will involve more evidence-based ratings on labels that will inform the consumer how effectively the cosmetic performs using standardized metrics [16].

Smooth sailing. If you are a middle-aged woman reading this book, chances are you have begun to show signs of age on your chest—I'm talking about those deep creases that develop between the breasts. Although some topical preparations may be effective for the shallow wrinkles on your face, you just won't find a cream that works well enough to alleviate wrinkles on this area of the body. Wrinkles on the chest can be caused by a bra that does not fit properly or by sleeping on your side. If you happen to be developing creases on your chest, try this simple test to determine if side sleeping is the cause. Lie on your side on your bed without wearing a bra. Allow your shoulders to collapse toward one another as if you were sleeping. Now, examine the area of skin between your breasts. If you see deep creases where the skin has folded in on itself, then creases on your chest will likely start to develop. Over time, these creases will become more pronounced and show even when you are not lying on your side.

The answer for chest creases is a clever new type of bra

designed to prevent this problem. Forget expensive "firming" creams. To reduce and prevent chest creases, you need to reduce the time that the skin between your breasts spends in a folded position. Designed to be worn at night, these bras are made without cups and usually without underwire. Instead of putting the support under the breasts, like a normal bra, these bras place support between the breasts. They position a semiflexible piece of foam or fabric between the breasts that prevents the breasts from falling on top of one another when sleeping in a side position. When the breasts are kept separated, the skin between them does not fold, and chest creases can be alleviated and even prevented. Using search terms like "chest wrinkle" and "bra," you can find many manufacturers of these awesome bras online.

Another item on the market for women is an antiwrinkle sticker for the chest. Shaped like a triangle and made using surgical adhesive, these stickers prevent the skin between the breasts from folding over on itself. Better for smaller-breasted women than the chest wrinkle bra, nightly use can significantly reduce the number of creases on the chest. However, because they are disposable, nightly use can make this product more expensive than the bra option.

Don't play with your food. Lately, there has been a great deal of buzz about calorie restriction as a method of achieving longevity. This latest craze is based on the research finding that reducing the number of calories fed to rats increased their life-span by 30 to 40 percent [17]. Calorie restriction has been shown to increase the average and maximum life-spans for several species [18]. One study even demonstrated complete prevention of age-related changes to the heart in mice [19]. Also for mice, calorie restriction showed protection against age-related neurological problems [20]. These findings suggest possible benefits of calorie restriction for age-related cognitive decline, memory loss, and dementia.

But what is the mysterious mechanism by which fewer calories lead to longer life? Theorists believe that reducing calories consumed reduces the production of free radicals and free radical-sourced aging [21]. (For a more complete discussion of the free radical theory of aging, see chapter 7.) Researchers have been able to observe that calorie-restricted rats exhibit less DNA damage from free radicals in major organs such as the heart, muscle, the brain, and the liver [22].

    What can we say about calorie restriction in humans? Unfortunately, science has not conducted enough clinical trials to say for sure whether this strategy works for us. The conditions to achieve this effect in animals are severe — animals only eat 50 to 70 percent of their daily diet to demonstrate efficacy. If you are thinking about trying this on yourself, consider that you have to reduce your current daily intake of food by almost half. People, that's a lot of iceberg lettuce. One trial on the rhesus monkey (an animal model closer to humans than mice and rats) has demonstrated a delay in disease onset and disease-related mortality under calorie restriction [23]. At the time of this publication, only one study was available suggesting a limited benefit of calorie restriction for humans [24]. Unfortunately, the degree of calorie restriction that you need to maintain to get the benefits may cause other problems along the way, such as severe body mass reduction and reduced ability to fight infection. It is hoped that this line of research will help us better understand the biochemical factors in the aging process so that new treatments based on the metabolic changes during calorie restriction can be implemented without starving the patient.

Get polarized. As we age, most of us begin to suffer from chronic aches and pains. Conversations about these ailments seem to take over the social interactions of older persons. We may also find that our propensity for injury goes up. I've even injured my back from lying on the couch for too long. As we age, more and more of our awareness is taken over by the physical experience of aches and pains. Many of us turn to powerful anti-inflammatory medications to cope with these changes in our bodies. But these medications come with their own set of risks and complications. If you happen to suffer from couch injuries like me, there is a nonpharmacological treatment that you can use at home to treat most kinds of muscle and joint strains. It's called magnet therapy. By applying a magnet of therapeutic strength to a pain-ridden muscle or joint, you can reduce your pain and speed healing. We will talk about why magnets help with these problems a little later. For now, let's review some clinical studies showing that magnets help with pain, mobility, and healing.

The use of magnets for pain and healing has recently exploded in the field of kinesiology. Studies showing the efficacy of magnets have employed the strongest type of experimental design: the double-blind study. In this experimental design, people with the same problems are assigned to a treatment group or a placebo group. The placebo group is given an inactive treatment that is similar enough to the active treatment to make them think that they are in the experimental group. For example, both groups are given treatment props that look like magnets; yet only one group receives an active magnet. Also, the researchers who interact with participants do not know who is receiving the experimental treatment and who is receiving the placebo treatment. This prevents subtle clues about group assignment from being passed along to participants from researchers who might have a vested interest in the findings. For example, were the study not double blinded, researchers who want magnets to come out on top might subtly encourage those in the active-magnet group to report more improvement than they actual experienced. With this check in place, any effect in the placebo group can be subtracted from the effect for the treatment group as a true measure of the power of the treatment. The following double-blind studies used some sort of fake magnet for half of the participants so that the researchers could isolate the effect of the real magnets on the other half of the group:

- *Magnets reduced knee pain and increased functional movement of the knee.* Patients with degenerative joint disease reported significant improvement following two weeks of magnet therapy [25].

- *Magnets improved disability and reduced pain.* Patients with chronic pelvic pain completed four weeks of treatment with magnets placed on abdominal trigger points [26].

- *Magnets reduced pain in the knee.* Patients with pain from osteoarthritis of the knee completed ten daily hours of magnet therapy for six weeks [27].

- *Magnets reduced menstrual pain.* Patients with regular dysmenorrhea were treated with a 2700 gauss magnet during the menstrual cycle. Reduced irritability was also suggested by the data [28].

- *Magnets reduced wrist pain and improved neuronal function.* Patients with carpal tunnel syndrome were administered a dynamic magnetic field to the wrist for four hours a day for two months [29].

In addition to these highly defined experimental studies, other researchers have reported pain reduction from magnetic bracelets [30], reduction in myofascial shoulder pain in patients with spinal cord injury [31], and a reduction in chronic lumbar radicular pain [32]. As you can see, the use of magnets has been linked to some amazing healing stories. But, to be fair, if you review the literature on magnet therapy, you will find an equal number of studies showing no effect for magnets. How do we reconcile these findings? Other authors have examined these "no effect" studies and concluded that the magnets used were not strong enough to provide therapeutic effect [33].

Even though we have clear research and anecdotal evidence that magnets are effective, we still do not have clear resolution on how they work. One theory is that magnets act on iron in the blood. When blood is exposed to a magnetic field, it causes a subtle movement and reorientation of red cells; this effect encourages blood flow to the magnetized area. With an increase in blood flow, the body can more easily clear fluid and swelling from the magnetized site. As swelling goes down, so does pressure on nerves. When pressure is reduced on nerves, pain goes down.

Unfortunately, you cannot make use of magnet therapy if you have a pacemaker, defibrillator, insulin pump, or other electrical device in your body. Magnets should also not be used after receiving steroid injections or with a transdermal drug patch. If you have any doubts about whether magnet therapy is contraindicated, speak with your medical provider.

Chapter 4

The Master Anti-aging Supplement

WHAT IF I TOLD YOU that you could use one supplement that would repair your skin, supercharge your immune system, build lean body mass, support healthy metabolism, attack viruses and bacteria directly, and accelerate your body's ability to heal from physical insults? This miracle supplement is nature's first food, a complex formula of compounds that Mother Nature has been perfecting for thousands of years. This chapter will share clinical research on using bovine colostrum as a topical cosmeceutical and as an oral neutraceutical to heal your entire body. It also offers a discussion on how this neutraceutical can boost the immune system and turn back the clock on the biological markers of aging.

The complexity and subtle inner workings of the body have great beauty when you look closely enough. This dance of atoms, molecules, and cells moves to the music of colostrum. Colostrum works on multiple systems of the body to return it to the level of function you had as a younger person. In this chapter, I offer clinical evidence to demonstrate how colostrum accomplishes all of these benefits for the body and has broad implications as an anti-aging supplement. If you are only going to choose a few of the anti-aging strategies I outline in this book, I hope that this healing food will be high on your list.

Laura Flynn Geissel, PhD

What Is Colostrum?

Colostrum is a master compound for the body, teaching it to perform at its peak. Where does it come from? When a mammal gives birth, a nutrient-rich fluid is produced by the mother prior to the production of milk. Colostrum is produced by the mother after birth for all mammals, including humans. If you are a woman who has had a child, you probably learned about the importance of colostrum from your doctor, midwife, or birthing class. It has been trumpeted worldwide by naturopaths, physicians, and natural healers to be an ancient anti-aging superfood. Colostrum is cutting-edge *and* ancient medicine for the body. Colostrum is cutting-edge because modern medicine has only recently begun to unlock its potential for human healing. Colostrum is the "new" miracle supplement because it has only been recently collected, processed, and packaged for adult human consumption. At the same time, colostrum is ancient because Mother Nature has been using it for hundreds of thousands of years to protect newborns and supercharge their development. Taken as an adult, it will turn back the clock on the entire body.

Colostrum is made up of the same compounds that we find naturally occurring in the body. Basically, Mother Nature took stock of all the compounds that the body needs to repair itself and fight off infection. Then she took all of these compounds and put them into mother's first milk—colostrum. Colostrum supercharges the body's own immune and repair system by increasing the bioavailability of your natural chemical triggers for defense and self-repair. If your mother nursed you as an infant, chances are that you have already taken colostrum.

Receiving colostrum as a newborn is a huge boost for proper development; we now know that receiving it is essential to the development of any newborn mammal. Colostrum provides immune, growth, and tissue repair factors that assist the newborn with growth and immunity. It contains antimicrobial agents that stimulate the development of the newborn's immune system. In addition to immune support, colostrum provides the newborn with amazing muscular-skeletal repair and growth capabilities [34].

Dr. Donald Henderson [35] at Sovereign Laboratories and the Center for Nutritional Research has made broad and exciting statements about the safety of colostrum and its usefulness:

> Only colostrum from dairy cows has been shown to be safe, natural, effective and biologically transferable for human use. Colostrum is a non-toxic, non-allergic food supplement that has no negative interactions with drugs, food, or other supplements. Bovine colostrum is not a drug. It is a safe, natural, non-allergenic food, taken by humans to treat and heal dozens of conditions—plus create new levels of vitality and well-being. . . . Bovine colostrum contains substances that are effective against many of the different microorganisms that are now resistant to the antibiotics on the market. . . . Colostrum is effective both as a treatment and a preventative measure for the immune system. It can prevent diseases and conditions such as colds, flu, diarrhea, sinusitis, asthma, allergies, herpes, viral bronchitis, candidiasis, and ear infections because it can boost underactive or weakened immune function. At the same time, it can also balance an overactive immune system, which is the situation for people who have an autoimmune disease (in which the body attacks its own healthy cells). When I first heard the claims about colostrum, I dismissed them. Now, after seeing the research and seeing patients' results for myself, I am a believer.

With expert medical testimony in hand, we can conclude that colostrum is one of the most important supplements you can take to maintain your health.

Lactoferrin, one of the main components of colostrum, has been extensively studied for its effect on the proper development of the newborn [36]. Specific receptor cells on the intestinal wall of the newborn collect and absorb colostrum. Lactoferrin helps the newborn to absorb important nutrients because it binds to metals (iron, manganese, and zinc) and brings them into the bloodstream of the baby when it is absorbed. Lactoferrin helps the endothelial cells in the gut reproduce and proliferate; this basically means that lactoferrin helps the stomach and intestine grow and meet the nutritional processing needs of the newborn. Lactoferrin also helps support the probiotic complement of the gut, suppressing the growth of pathogenic bacteria while promoting the growth of friendly bacteria such as lactobacillus and bifidobacterium. Finally, colostrum contains numerous compounds that both support and educate the infant's immune system in its transition from dependence on the mother to independence. By extension, you can reap many of these benefits by taking colostrum as an adult. As you turn the pages of this chapter, you will learn much more about how this amazing superfood can benefit an adult's body.

You may be thinking to yourself, "That all sounds great, but I'm not going to drink breast milk to get it." No problem. (Whew!) Another miraculous thing about colostrum is that this fluid is replaceable across mammals. That means that cow colostrum is as effective for humans as human colostrum. Today, you can now find many topical and capsule formulations of colostrum that have been collected from cows to assist in maintaining your good health. Colostrum in powder form looks and tastes a lot like powdered milk. Humans can achieve a diversity of rich benefits by supplementing with bovine sources of colostrum [37]. Not all colostrum products are made the same; we will talk about what science says to look for in a colostrum product in chapter 5.

The discovery of colostrum and its effects on infant and adult health has been truly remarkable. Researchers have isolated all of the main components of this special substance that contribute to overall health. In the 2005 edition of the *Gale Encyclopedia of Alternative Medicine,* Rebecca Frey, PhD, and Teresa Odle [38] provided a list of the major components of colostrum and their benefits. I have reprinted the list here so that you can get an overview of these benefits. We will deal with these compounds individually as you work through this chapter:

Immunoglobulins. Immunoglobulins are globulin proteins that function as antibodies. They are the most plentiful immune factors found in colostrum. Immunoglobulin G (IgG) counteracts bacteria and toxins in the blood and lymphatic system; immunoglobulin M (IgM) seeks out and attaches itself to viruses in the circulatory system; immunoglobulin D and E (IgD and IgE) remove foreign substances from the bloodstream and activate allergic reactions. High-quality colostrum is certified to contain a minimum of 16% immunoglobulins.

Lactoferrin. Lactoferrin is a protein that transports iron to red blood cells and helps to deprive viruses and harmful bacteria of iron.

Proline-rich polypeptide (PRP). PRP is a hormone that regulates the thymus gland, helping to calm a hyperactive immune system or stimulate an underactive immune system.

Growth factors. The growth factors in bovine colostrum include insulin-like growth factors (IGF-1 and IGF-2), an epithelial growth factors (EGF), transforming growth factors (TgF-A and TgF-B), and a platelet-derived growth factor (PDGF). Growth factors stimulate normal growth as well as the healing and repair of aged or injured skin, muscle, and other tissues. In addition, growth factors help the body to burn fat instead of muscle for fuel when a person is dieting for fasting.

Growth hormone. Growth hormone slows some signs of aging.

Leukocytes. Leukocytes are white blood cells that stimulate production of interferon, a protein that inhibits viruses from reproducing.

Enzymes. Colostrum contains three enzymes that oxidize (help to kill) bacteria.

Cytokines and lymphokines. These are substances that regulate the body's immune response, stimulate the production of immunoglobulins, and affect cell growth and repair.

Vitamins. Colostrum contains small amounts of vitamins A, B, and E.

Glycoproteins. Glycoproteins, or protease inhibitors, are complex proteins that protect immune factors and growth factors from being broken down by the acids in the digestive tract.

Sulfur. Sulfur is a mineral that is an important building block of proteins.

How Science Opened Its Arms to Colostrum

Colostrum has a long history of study for its immune system boosting properties. Even though the potential for colostrum to be front-line medicine against illness was well documented as early as the 1980s, it seems like medical science went down a different road. Rather than focusing on putting the body's own healing mechanisms to better use during illness, medical science turned its attention to pharmaceuticals that would do the work of the immune system. Unfortunately, the usefulness of certain classes of pharmaceuticals, like antibiotics, is beginning to wane as more and more infections become drug resistant. And let's not even get into the very serious side effects that accompany most medications on the market.

Now, we are experiencing a sea change in medical science. Modern medicine has realized that modern diseases are getting worse in severity and are more prevalent than ever before. When was the last time modern medicine actually cured a disease? Doctors need a new kind of medicine to heal the pathogenic challenges of the modern world. Medical science is now investigating ways to better use people's own healing processes to manage disease. For example, some exciting new cancer research is under way in which the cancer patient's own white blood cells are removed from the body, modified, and put back into the patient to attack the tumor. As medical science has turned its attention to better understanding the immune system and the methods for using the body's own healing machinery, there has been renewed interest in colostrum for treatment-resistant diseases.

In 1990, we learned that an immunoglobulin preparation could be made from colostrum [39]. This preparation had a high antibacterial antibody titer and a very strong ability to neutralize bacterial toxins. (One of the things that make us feel so bad during a bacterial infection is the complex group of toxins that bacteria put into the body.) These researchers described the colostrum preparation as well tolerated and highly effective in the treatment of infectious diarrhea. By 1995, the scientific literature had concluded that colostrum was bactericidal against *Helicobacter pylori* [40] and could also kill certain protozoans such as *Cryptosporidium parvum* [41].

Also by this time, a fascinating study on passive immunization of children with bovine colostrum had been conducted [42]. This study showed that cows who had developed an immunity to a virus could pass on this immunity to humans through oral administration of bovine colostrum. The virus under study in the children was rotavirus, a type of virus that infects the intestinal tract, causing diarrhea. This virus is one of the main reasons that infants and young children are admitted to the hospital; in short, it's a huge problem for young, developing immune systems. Infants admitted to the hospital for other reasons are highly vulnerable to acquiring this virus from their sick peers. In the study we are discussing, researchers inoculated twenty-five pregnant Freisian cows with a vaccine containing all four human rotaviruses. They then studied about one hundred children admitted to the hospital by giving half of them colostrum from the cows who had given birth and the other half an artificial infant formula. In this study, 14 percent of the children receiving the artificial infant formula contracted rotavirus while in the hospital, yet *none* of the children who had received passive immunization against rotavirus through orally administered colostrum got sick. These kids took some pills of colostrum, got no side effects, and stayed well. These findings were a huge step forward in building the case that the immune factors from cow colostrum could be passed along to humans and improve their health.

Today, research on colostrum is accelerating. We know that receiving colostrum is essential to the developing immune system of any mammal [43]. We also know that colostrum helps the immune system defeat viruses, bacteria, and fungi. For example, colostrum can neutralize endotoxins arising from gram-negative bacteria and inhibits reactions to these toxins in animal model studies [44]. Clinical trials with bovine colostrum show that it reduces the influx of endotoxins into the bloodstream from the gut; this may be a major mechanism underlying its therapeutic effect against gram-negative bacteria. Not only does colostrum reduce serum endotoxins but it also reduces inflammatory markers that we usually see with endotoxin exposure.

In this section, we have shown how interest in colostrum has increased in recent years. Next, we talk in more detail about how you can use colostrum to freeze the hands of that biological clock you worry so much about.

Colostrum and Anti-aging Support

One of the reasons that we experience aging is that our natural physical repair mechanisms decline in efficacy as we get older. For example, when human growth hormone levels drop with age, the body experiences a reduction in its ability to heal and regulate itself. Remember, cells all over the body are aging and dying every second. These cells must be replaced, and the rate at which they are replaced is controlled by the growth hormone feedback loops in the body. One of the most important growth hormones is human growth hormone (HGH). Through natural chemical processes in the body, the presence of HGH leads to the creation of a workhorse compound called insulin-like growth factor (IGF). So, although HGH is one of the most important growth hormones in the body, most of its work is done through two growth factors called IGF-1 and IGF-2.

HGH is most prevalent in the body during childhood. It is very important in regulating the growth of children—too much and the child will be too tall, and too little will result in a growth delay. When we hit adulthood, the production of HGH declines and continues to decline as we age. This means that the body has less available HGH to maintain health, and its decline brings about aging. HGH helps the body to maintain heart health, physical stamina, muscle strength, kidney flow, physical temperature, and metabolic rate. When HGH declines because of aging, all of these systems begin to suffer. Because IGF is the workhorse of HGH, we can measure it over the lifespan to surmise the activity level of our innate growth factors. As women reach middle age, their HGH levels can drop by up to 70 percent as compared to their youthful peers.

By using colostrum to restore our natural levels of growth hormones, we can return to youthful efficiency in cell repair. Colostrum may not contain high levels of HGH, but it is a huge source of IGF-1—one of the most vital components of colostrum [45]. Growth factors are proteins that control cell growth and how fast your body performs basic chemical conversions like converting glucose into energy. They help cells in the hormone, immune, and neurological system talk to one another and coordinate regeneration and repair. The growth factor called IGF-1 enters cells to do repair work and stimulates cell growth where the body needs it most [46]. When we replace our declining levels of growth factors with a colostrum supplement, we dramatically change the body's resilience. For example, increasing levels of IGF leads to increased tissue repair. In this study, local IGF-1 was administered to a group of wounded animals. Those given IGF-1 showed significant gains in lean body weight and bone regrowth [47]. The researchers also proposed that local administration of IGF-1 could have significant positive implications for the repair of peripheral nerves. If your body could be considered "vintage," colostrum can provide you with a steady supply of your own innate repair mechanisms.

Colostrum Rebuilds the Immune System

Colostrum rebuilds the immune system and helps the body fight off infections of all kinds. If I ran out of money to buy colostrum, I would mortgage the house to get more. The stuff has just been that good for my overall health. Now, I'd like to focus on colostrum as an immune modulator. If your immune system just isn't working as well as it used to, or if you just want to increase your resistance to disease, then colostrum can really help you. This compound can also help an overactive immune system figure out when to relax. The following pages go over some of the best clinical research on the effects of colostrum on the immune system.

Taking colostrum as an anti-aging supplement gives you the very pleasant effect of a supercharged immune system. What if someone told you that you could enroll in an experimental study to test a new drug that would multiply the strength of your immune system and restore your resilience? Would you sign up? I'll bet that you would seriously consider it. Luckily for us, Mother Nature has been running this same experiment on mammals for hundreds of thousands of years. The result is a perfect healing food that you can take without a prescription. The multiple impacts of colostrum on the immune system come from the presence of a few different compounds. Colostrum does not add anything foreign to the body; its mission is to increase the bioavailability of the compounds that your own body uses during an immune response. The active compounds in colostrum include (1) immune system activators, (2) compounds that interfere directly with the activity of invaders such as bacteria and viruses, and (3) basic building blocks of the immune system.

First, colostrum provides the body with more of the chemical messengers that it uses to regulate the activity of the immune system. These triggers, such as cytokines, lymphokines, and PRP, tell the immune system when to turn on. They also tell the body when to make immunoglobulins, the basic functional unit of the immune system. Second, colostrum includes compounds that directly attack invading bacteria and viruses. Colostrum interacts with them in ways that limit their growth and ability to infect cells. These colostrum-derived compounds include enzymes and a truly magical protein called lactoferrin. Additionally, colostrum provides the body with a ready supply of compounds that form the basic foot soldiers of the immune system. All of the immunoglobulins in colostrum play a role in traveling through the body on invader search-and-destroy missions. Each immunoglobulin in colostrum plays a slightly different, yet important, role in protecting the body.

The main immunoglobulins found in mammary secretions are IgG, IgA, and IgM. This molecule is essentially one long strand of amino acids (a protein) that rolls up into a ball when placed in a water-based environment. The manner in which the protein rolls up into a ball, or "glob," forms an active site that interacts chemically with other compounds to accomplish a task. The "Ig" stands for immunoglobulin, while the third letter identifies the type of immunoglobulin that corresponds to function. When we are first exposed to a foreign body or invader, IgM is the class of immunoglobulins that the body first mobilizes. IgM is basically a first responder to an infection. IgA is the major type of immunoglobulin that is found in mucosal secretions. When your nose is running, the mucus contains an immunoglobulin that helps to defeat pathogens before they get a chance to enter the body and infect cells. IgG is a class of generalized immunoglobulins that are the main class found in colostrum and milk [48]. In fact, colostrum has a huge amount of these proteins; the immunoglobulin levels in colostrum are a hundred times greater than what is found in actual milk [49].

Finally, colostrum contains a small number of natural killer cells. Natural killer cells are a type of lymphocyte that the body makes to attack invaders at about three days after infection. Approximately 0.5 percent of all colostral cells are natural killer cells that your body can put to work [50]. When you consume a serving of colostrum, you get all of that immune support wrapped up in another set of compounds that protect it from the stomach acid (glycoproteins). These compounds increase absorption through the digestive tract.

I've just given you a broad overview of how colostrum boosts the immune system. How does the cow develop the immune factors that are passed along in colostrum? Insights into this process have been provided by Doug Wyatt at the Center of Nutritional Research [51]:

> Bovine colostrum contains hundreds of thousands of antibodies, so many that we should consider the cow a "walking pharmaceutical factory." These antibodies develop within twenty-four hours of a cow coming into contact with a pathogen (i.e. pathogens in the soil, air, feed, or from human contact), and are subsequently passed into colostrum and milk. . . . Colostrum has been found to contain specific antibodies to more than nineteen specific disease-causing pathogens including: E

coli, salmonella, candida, streptococcus, staphylococcus, H. pylori, cryptosporidium, and rotavirus.

So the basic scenario here is that the cow is exposed to many of the same pathogens that affect humans. The cow then develops immunity that can be passed along to its offspring. By taking that colostrum as an oral supplement, this same immunity is conferred to you. This is what a practicing, Johns Hopkins-trained, board-certified physician had to say about the clinical usefulness of colostrum [52]:

> I prescribe colostrum to about one third of my patients. The anecdotal evidence shows that patients are thriving after taking the supplement—that their conditions usually improve substantially. And if we can help the patient get better without standard drugs, we do it. I think the new cutting-edge nutritional biochemistry is very exciting—and that includes colostrum. The factors found in colostrum work together to enhance the immune system. . . . When I discovered colostrum, I confirmed that it had been extensively studied by highly reputable doctors, scientists, and organizations.

Scientists have actually broken down the immune response into its component parts to investigate where colostrum has the greatest impact [53]. By monitoring the blood of people who were given orally administered colostrum, scientific observations included an increase in the types of cells the body uses to attack invaders. These new natural killer cells were mobilized into circulating blood within two hours after ingesting colostrum. As these increases were shown to revert to normal levels within a few hours, these findings lend support to taking colostrum in divided doses throughout the day.

But what about people with suppressed immune systems? People can present with compromised immune function from a variety of causes ranging from autoimmune diseases to HIV and

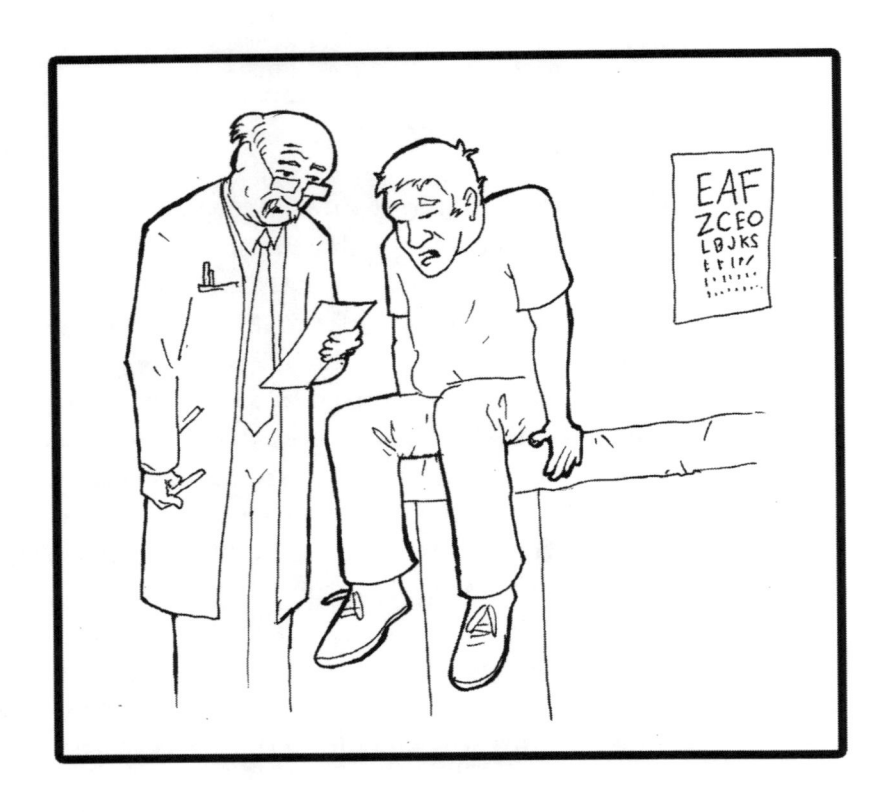

"Doc, I think I have chronic fatigue syndrome."
"Yeah, you and one billion other people."

medications with immune suppression as a side effect. One of the problems with cancer treatment is that chemotherapy wipes out the immune system. Because your body needs a functioning immune system to discover and destroy cancerous cells, this has always been a controversy with this type of treatment. This immunosuppressant effect is also present to a degree with antibiotics, though to a much lesser extent than with chemotherapy. Azithromycin may kill bacteria in the sinuses, but it also slows down your immune system at the same time by reducing the efficiency of your mitochondria in producing energy for the cell. Wouldn't it be great if we had a compound that would counteract immune suppression?

To investigate the potential benefits of colostrum in restoring a suppressed immune system, researchers created a group of mice with artificially suppressed immune systems. They administered a sublethal dose of cyclophosphamide that was shown to reduce the antibody-forming cells in the spleen. So now we have a group of chemically suppressed immune systems that provides an animal model of chemotherapy. These mice were given bovine lactoferrin in their drinking water for five weeks. They exhibited a seven- to tenfold increase in spleen antibody-forming cells as compared to mice who were not given lactoferrin. We can conclude that prolonged, oral administration of lactoferrin for chemically immunocompromised mice leads to the partial restoration of the immune response [54]. These findings would seem to have direct implications for patients whose immune systems had been suppressed through chemical means like chemotherapy.

The research we have covered so far illustrates the ability of colostrum to boost the immune system, making it more efficient and harder working. But colostrum not only amplifies the immune system, it can also help an overactive immune system to calm down [55]. One of the main components of colostrum, a group of PRP, acts as a messenger chemical for the immune system. PRP tells the cells in the immune system when to make immunoglobulins that are used as antibodies to fight off infection. PRP also tells the immune system when to make helper T cells and when to make suppressor T cells. John Buhmeyer at the Center for Nutritional Research described in detail how PRP regulates the immune system [55]:

> PRP acts as a hormone in the thymus gland by stimulating thymocytes (lymphocytes that originated in the thymus gland) to differentiate and become activated as either helper or suppressor T cells. Helper T cells present foreign antigen (such as a protein from a virus or bacteria) to B cells, lymphocytes which originate in the bone marrow and which produce antibodies that are specific to the antigens presented to them by the helper T cells. . . . Suppressor T cells, on the other hand, deactivate other lymphocytes to "turn off" the immune response after an infection is under control. This is important because if the response is not turned off, normal tissue will be damaged. Autoimmune diseases, such as rheumatoid arthritis, lupus or diabetes Type 1, are characterized by overactive immune systems that attack the tissues of the body. PRP has shown promise against autoimmune diseases in preliminary trials.

As we collect more and more information about colostrum, it certainly sounds like it is good for whatever ails us. One study conducted in Africa with HIV/AIDS patients administered an oral PRP spray every four hours to participants. Over a ninety-day period, participants exhibited a remarkable decrease in viral counts as a clinically significant increase in CD4+ lymphocytes. Symptoms of diarrhea, vomiting, cough, tuberculosis, and paresthesia were eradicated for treated participants. Thanks to the miracle of the PRP in colostrum, these patients were able to enjoy a higher quality of life with no side effects from the treatment [56].

Finally, I'll tell you a personal story about how colostrum

healed the health of my seven-year-old niece. Winter is always a difficult time in my sister's house; she has two school-aged children who bring home every disease known to man. This winter had been particularly difficult for my young niece; and doctors had proclaimed it one of the worst cold and flu seasons on record. Sienna was constantly going to the doctor and being prescribed multiple rounds of antibiotics. Eventually, they just did not know what else to do for her to make her well again. Her cough had persisted for six weeks, and it was so severe that she could never get to sleep. All the doctors could say was, "Well, her lungs are really strong." What does that even mean, "her lungs are really strong"? That is what a doctor says when he doesn't really know what is wrong but feels like he has to say something! I finally told my sister that it was time to start Sienna on colostrum. We put her on one to two teaspoons of the power (in ice cream) per day. Within a few days, she began to have improvement, and her persistent cough dried up in a week without having to take more antibiotics. Since then, Sienna made it through the rest of the school year without catching any new colds. Thanks to the miracle of colostrum, her health is back on track. Since Sienna is not bringing home as many infections, the health of the whole household has improved for the better.

COLOSTRUM AND PERFORMANCE ENHANCEMENT

Colostrum is a nutritional supplement that can help you achieve peak performance in any sport. Peak performance is when you are functioning at your absolute personal best in the athletic activity of your choosing. It's when the division between the mind and body disappears and you *are* the movement. Peak performance is an attitude for physical achievement that reinforces reaching to the very limit of our ability with every game, run, or workout. The notion of peak performance came out of psychology. It developed from the perspective that what we believe we can do is the best predictor of what we actually will do. If I believe that I am going to burn more calories with this workout than I ever have before, then I am more likely to actually do it. Peak performance has also been applied to business and helps executives achieve their topmost performance.

Peak performance involves an emotional state that predisposes to top physical performance. But my ability to achieve my best as an athlete also depends on physical readiness. I can have all the positive beliefs about my ability in the world, but if my body isn't prepared to work, then I am unlikely to run that three minute mile. Using colostrum as a neutraceutical both prepares the body for physical performance and assists the body in recovering more quickly after the stress of exercise. Put all of that together with a peak performance attitude about your ability and you'll be a winner every time.

People who care about helping people maximize their physical effectiveness have investigated the impact of colostrum on physiological processes. One study took a group of active men and women who were assigned heavy-resistance and aerobic training three times a week. Using an eight-week training program, these participants were divided into a whey protein supplementation group and a colostrum group (twenty grams a day of colostrum). When the performance of the colostrum group was compared to the whey protein group, the former showed significantly greater increases in lean body mass at eight weeks [57]. If you are into exercise, you know that lean body mass means putting on muscle, not fat. So the colostrum group bulked up with muscle. If you are interested in putting on muscle to enhance your physical readiness (or just to look good), you might consider adding twenty grams of colostrum to your diet during intensive training.

Colostrum is big news. In fact, there is an entire institute devoted to colostrum research; you can do some of your own investigation about the miracle of colostrum at ColostrumResearch.org. When I looked through the research done by the institute, I found some wonderful papers on the use of colostrum for peak physical performance. What are some of the active ingredients in colostrum that are so beneficial to athletes? It is believed that the contribution to athletic performance has to do with the growth factors in colostrum, such as IGF-1. These growth factors basically stimulate the body to grow and repair damaged tissues.

If you know your exercise physiology, you know that effective strenuous exercise actually causes microtears and other sorts of tissue stress. It is the body's repair of these microtears that builds up the muscle to make it better able to handle the same level of work (or stress) in the future. If you have additional growth factors on board, such as IGF-1, then there is a positive effect on muscle rebuilding during and after training [58]. These growth factors can help the muscle repair more quickly after exercise that causes microtears. Finally, researchers conducted a review of many studies investigating the impact of bovine colostrum on exercise performance. In their review, they concluded that the addition of bovine colostrum to the diet is most effective during periods of highly intense training and recovery from intense training. They proposed that the effect is due to elevated IGF-I, improved intramuscular buffering capacity, an increase in lean body mass, and an increase in salivary IgA [59].

Are you a runner? Running is a convenient and popular form of exercise. You don't need any equipment or a gym membership; simply with some shoes and the clothes on your back, you can get a great workout. If you want to be able to run farther and harder, then colostrum is for you. Folks at the Center for Research in Education and Sports Science conducted a study on running and colostrum supplementation. This research hits the nail on the head for what colostrum can really do for the body in a performance context. In this study, thirty-nine men completed an eight-week running program while consuming sixty grams a day of bovine colostrum or a placebo of whey protein. To test performance at weeks 0, 4, and 8, subjects were placed on a treadmill and instructed to keep running until they were exhausted. During the first phase of the running program, no considerable differences in performance were observed for the two groups. All participants showed an increase in distance covered on the treadmill for the first four weeks. (Training does work!) But in the last four weeks, the colostrum group continued to improve, while the whey protein group plateaued on the treadmill test. In sum, participants in the colostrum group ran farther and were able to exert themselves more on a treadmill test with increasing grade [60].

Colostrum really has the potential to help runners attain their distance and endurance training goals. How does colostrum do this for runners? The growth factor in colostrum (IGF-1) probably helped runners in the experimental group to repair and increase lean muscle mass as a result of training. That means that taking colostrum and sitting on the couch is not going to increase muscle mass or your endurance. It is the interaction between strenuous exercise and the growth factors in colostrum that increases muscle mass and leads to enhanced performance. Colostrum builds muscle by working hard on those little microtears and builds bigger muscles from these repair efforts. Without microtears, there is nothing for colostrum to repair, and muscles will not be enhanced. Finally, another clinical study has shown that the presence of IGF-1 promotes muscle protein synthesis — more IGF-1 on board from colostrum facilitates the growth of lean muscle mass [61].

Colostrum and Skin Repair

You are reading this book because you want to look and feel younger. Not only does colostrum heal your insides, it also heals you on the outside. The future of skin care is going to involve a strategic combination of cosmeceuticals and nutraceuticals to reverse the biological aging process and degenerative skin changes [62]. This means that a combination of topical compounds and orally dispensed nutrients will give us the best chance of looking ageless. Bovine colostrum liberates the body from the visual, inflammatory, and hormonal markers of aging. This compound is an all-natural cosmeceutical that will ease away your wrinkles and improve the overall quality and health of your skin. When used as a neutraceutical, this supplement is so beneficial that it boosts your immune system while reinventing your skin at the same time. Ask yourself, "How much money do I spend a year on wrinkle creams?" What if I could recommend a product to you that costs less than fancy skin creams, works better for healing skin, and has an overall positive effect on your general health? Colostrum heals the body on the inside, and then this supercharged inner health radiates out through the skin.

Colostrum will reinvent your skin. When used topically, colostrum acts on the skin like a cosmeceutical, repairing the skin from the outside in. This compound will heal the skin where it is applied. When taken internally, colostrum acts like a neutraceutical, nourishing and repairing the skin from the inside out. If you want the skin over your entire body to look and feel better, consider colostrum as an oral supplement. Its healing magic of innate chemical messengers is absorbed through the digestive tract and delivered to the skin. If there is an area of the body that you want to target for skin repair, such as the face or décolleté, you may use colostrum as a topical cosmeceutical. Either way, the right dose or application of colostrum is a powerful anti-aging tool. Incorporating this miracle substance into your daily health regimen will take years off your face, or any other area of the skin on which you use it. I initially healed my skin by taking the supplement as an oral neutraceutical. But the literature review that I conducted says that you can get the same (or better) effect from a targeted application with a topical cream. When my skin needs a little extra help, I add in the topical application for the extra repair factors. This supplement is a perfect blend of topical and internal healing; together, they reduce the clinical signs of aging for the skin.

How does colostrum improve the health of your skin? Your skin has the built-in repair mechanisms that it needs to be beautiful and healthy. Colostrum simply acts to correct the decline in our natural repair systems as we age. Colostrum just returns the level of the body's functionality to a younger state. Now let's talk about how these compounds work synergistically to give you younger skin. The single most important factor in the ability of colostrum to reverse the signs of visible (and invisible) aging is the presence of epidermal growth factor (EGF) [63]. You can think of this growth factor like a skin repair messenger that tells your skin cells to heal. Colostrum is the only supplement or cosmeceutical that includes innate growth factors for healing the skin. This is the only "wrinkle cream" on the market that uses the repair factors that nature made, not ones synthesized in a lab. This supplement will not only improve the visual appearance of your skin but will also heal your skin from the inside out.

Colostrum has a titanic amount of EGF as compared to any other substance on the planet. EGF can repair skin damage owing to normal healthy aging and aging resulting from environmental damage from sun, chemicals, or injuries. This is because the growth factors in colostrum tell your skin cells to rev up their engines, repair themselves, and more quickly replace old layers of skin with new ones. This is the same principle underlying Retin-A or retinol-type skin care products. So when I told you that the master anti-aging supplement would heal your skin from the inside out, I am talking about its ability to up-regulate skin repair. In fact, elasticity returns to the skin while taking colostrum, thus reducing the appearance of fine lines and wrinkles. Over time, these growth factors can assist in repair and regeneration throughout the entire body.

Dermatologists have conducted lots of research on the healing benefits of colostrum for the skin. For example, one study showed that applying a topical colostrum cream to scar tissue resulted in a reduction of scar tissue and a smoother visual appearance [64]. Other researchers have looked at specific types of skin cells and applied colostrum to them in a petri dish. They found that the application of colostrum promoted the growth and replication of these cells through the activation of tyrosine kinase receptors [65]. There have also been some solid research studies demonstrating that isolating the EFG from colostrum and applying it to the skin can have a miraculous effect on the skin's healing ability. The department of surgery at a VA medical center in Washington, D.C., investigated the effect of EGF on wound healing [66]. As wound healing is a major concern for departments of surgery, they were highly motivated to better understand this process. A ten-day study of cultured epithelial cells was used by researchers to demonstrate the relationship between EGF and skin healing. EGF was shown to stimulate DNA synthesis on days 3 and 7 of the study. (DNA synthesis is an indicator of new skin growth.) Each batch of skin cells exposed to EGF also exhibited something called epidermal outgrowth—basically the same thing as epithelial regeneration from a wound edge. Of all the different growth factors investigated in the study, EGF was responsible for the greatest regeneration of cells. So using some logic called the transitive property, we can write a simple equation:

If EGF = Skin Regeneration
AND
Colostrum = EGF
THEN
Colostrum = Skin Regeneration
DONE.

In addition to helping your skin look younger, colostrum also protects it from certain diseases. Another component of colostrum, lactoferrin, works as a general stimulant of the immune system and can target existing or developing tumor vasculature. Lactoferrin has shown clinical activity against skin melanoma with low toxicity [67]. This means that lactoferrin is a potent compound for preventing the formation of cancerous skin tumors and for attacking tumors that are already formed. So if you happen to be one of those people who had overexposure to the sun, you may be concerned about the possibility of developing skin cancer during your lifetime. Growing up, I remember my stay-at-home mother languishing in the sun every summer. If you were wondering where Mom was, the first place to check was the lawn chair in the backyard. Today, she has had multiple small surgeries on her face to remove precancerous lesions.

Even if you use sun block religiously, there is always skin damage associated with UV radiation. Some UV radiation always gets past these blocks. If you have read the label on your bottle of sun block, you may remember that it says to reapply every two hours. Know anyone who follows this direction? Also, know that there is no such thing as a healthy tan. I hate to have to tell you this, but any change in skin color means too much exposure to UV radiation. Your body is trying to prevent this level of exposure by increasing the melanin in the skin. If you see a tan come up, it is too late; the UV radiation has penetrated to the deeper layers of the skin. The reason that the skin on our faces gets wrinkled as we age is that facial skin suffers the most damage from sun exposure.

If you want to know how much exposure to the sun has affected the skin on your face, compare the quality of your facial skin to the quality of the skin on your chest. I imagine you will see a huge difference in thickness, texture, and moisture. If you observe any significant difference, then you could significantly benefit from a trial of colostrum to repair the sun-damaged skin. When we were kids, my parents loved the beach. We would head out to Ocean City, Maryland, a couple times a month every summer. Being fair skinned and blue eyed, I came home every weekend looking like a cooked beet, with sunburn so hot and red that I couldn't even sleep. Thanks to colostrum, you would never know that my skin suffered this abuse as a young person. I sincerely believe that the only reason I haven't had precancerous lesions like my mother is my consistent use of colostrum to prevent abnormal cell changes.

Personal success stories in using colostrum for the skin. I began taking colostrum when I was first ill with Lyme disease. I was thirty-seven at the time, and my skin was beginning to show the first signs of aging. About a month after starting on bovine colostrum, I noticed my energy and resistance to respiratory illnesses seemed to be improving. I had always been very vulnerable to colds and flus, so this was a pleasant surprise. Also, I started to feel more positive about my appearance when I looked in the mirror. Being a behavioral scientist by training, I told myself that this was wishful thinking and that my skin was no different than it had been a month ago. But as the months went by, I became more youthful in appearance. My skin now looks better at forty than it did when I was thirty. People who don't know me consistently think I'm in my twenties.

I recently recommended colostrum to my friend Jeff, who had been caught in a house fire. One day, one of the space heaters upstairs caught fire. In an attempt to save the house, Jeff tried to move a burning area rug with his hands. He saved the house but suffered severe burns on both hands. After a trip to the emergency room and a consult with the burn unit, Jeff returned home on pain pills and with both hands bandaged. He was told by the doctors that he would have scars on his hands for the rest of his life. When I heard about his burns, I contacted him and told him about colostrum, its effect on my skin, and the research I had done on it. I talked him into taking it for his burns, and he has never regretted it. Every time he returned to the clinic for follow-up, the nurses and doctors were amazed at how well his skin was healing. To the amazement of his doctors, his hands healed perfectly with no scars.

A Healing Supplement for the Whole Body

The perfect soup of healing compounds in colostrum has a diverse effect on multiple organ systems of the body. This section reviews some of the research on colostrum for healing some of the most common health challenges that we all face. Keep in mind that information in this section is very technical. I have gone to great lengths to find medical research from the scientific community that validates the healing qualities of the miracle supplement. Feel free to read those sections that have the most implications for your life and the people in it. For example, if you happen to have an inflammatory bowel disease or know someone who does, then read the section on defending the gut. If this type of disorder has no context in your life, go ahead and skip that section. Think of this chapter like an encyclopedia on colostrum.

Colostrum dropkicks bacteria and fungi. In 1949, a man named Sherwood Lawrence discovered molecules that he called *transfer factors*. While treating tuberculosis (TB), he found that immune response to TB could be induced by transferring blood from one patient to another. Once transferred, these immune factors educated the recipient's immune system to fight off TB. Bovine colostrum happens to be one of the most abundant sources of transfer factors that is known by medical science. The transfer factors in colostrum include immunoglobulins like IgG. In sum, the transfer factors in colostrum make it an ideal weapon against invading bacteria, viruses, and fungi. Studies have shown that colostrum kills *E. coli, Candida albicans,* rotaviruses, and cryptosporidium [35]. Using this knowledge, makers of colostrum have exposed cows to invasive yeast (*C. albicans*) to increase the fungi-fighting ability of the colostrum that is passed on to the newborn. You can even purchase colostrum that has enhanced transfer factors specific to yeast. The future of medical research may reveal cures for many childhood diseases that come from targeted enhancements to colostrum.

Could this miracle supplement become the next generation of antibiotic therapy? It's really exciting to consider this possibility! The antimicrobial elements of colostrum include lactoferrin, lysozyme, lactoperoxidase, and immunoglobulins [61]. The body uses this complex soup of enzymes and proteins to fight off invaders. Colostrum is well populated with immunoglobulins, and we can use these compounds to make agents of the immune system that go out on seek-and-destroy missions for the body.

Lactoferrin has demonstrated antibacterial properties in vitro [68] and in vivo [69]. It's very easy for a compound to demonstrate antibiotic properties in a culture or test tube (*in vitro*). It is much more difficult to demonstrate clinical effectiveness against a bacterium in a living animal or person (*in vivo*). Colostrum passes both tests.

Many compounds that kill bacteria in a petri disk also kill the host when administered at levels necessary for clinical effectiveness. For example, bleach kills streptococcus (strep throat) very effectively in a test tube, but you cannot really drink it for your throat. So the tricky part is finding a compound that will kill bacteria and viruses without killing the person. The fact that lactoferrin has demonstrated in vivo antibiotic properties is huge. When I saw my first doctor for Lyme disease, he told me an interesting fact about antibiotics. Left alone, without any help from the body's immune system, a person would have to take antibiotics for a year to kill off a strep throat infection. That's a long time. More important, it highlights the power of your immune system at work; we only need to take a seven- to ten-day course of antibiotics to kill off strep throat. That means that what does most of the work to eradicate infection is actually your own immune system.

Lactoferrin kills bacteria according to two mechanisms. First, this protein has a bacteriostatic effect on invading bacteria. *Bacteriostatic* essentially means that lactoferrin inhibits the reproduction and spread of the bacteria so that the body's own immune system can get on top of the infection. Lactoferrin is a dominant binder of iron, and this deprives bacteria (that require iron) of a very essential nutrient. In fact, this protein can slow down the growth of any micro-organism that requires iron, including gram-negative bacteria, gram-positive bacteria, and certain types of yeast [68,70,71]. The second mechanism of lactoferrin activity is bactericidal, meaning that this protein actually kills bacteria with which it comes into contact. At concentrations found within the body, lactoferrin damages the cell wall of gram-negative bacteria by stimulating the release of lipopolysaccharides.

Finally, there is evidence to support the hypothesis that lactoferrin can have a preventative activity against infection. In one study, mice were administered lactoferrin intravenously (through an IV drip) and intraperitoneally (through injection into the body cavity). These mice were then given a lethal dose of *E. coli* using both administration methods (IV drip and injection). These mice survived as a result of the antibacterial effects of lactoferrin [72,73]. So, by taking a lactoferrin supplement before we get sick, we can better prepare the body with the resources it needs when illness strikes.

Colostrum punches out viruses. Everyone reading this book has dealt with a virus at one time or another. Viruses span the continuum of severity from the common cold to HIV. Whether you are dealing with an acute, short-lived virus like a respiratory infection or a serious, chronic infection like hepatitis, research shows that colostrum can help. One of the main components of colostrum, lactoferrin, has been studied extensively for its antiviral properties. In fact, practically every study shows that it is fantastic at inhibiting virus proliferation and at assisting the body in reducing its viral load. But don't take my word for it — let's take a look at some of the research on this topic.

One of the ways that researchers develop a case for the efficacy of colostrum is to examine people with a particular disorder and profile the chemical defense and repair triggers that are associated with that disorder. For example, people with allergic skin conditions display more lactoferrin in their skin than people with normal skin. People with inflammatory conditions of the bowel display more lactoferrin in the digestive tract than people without these conditions. Fundamentally, an increase in lactoferrin means that the body is producing extra in an attempt to heal itself. It has been found that lactoferrin production increases from four up to two hundred micrograms per milliliter during microbial infections and autoimmune disease [74]. By profiling different diseases by what chemical triggers the body uses to manage them, we can strategize ways to increase levels of these chemicals and supercharge the body.

Using this line of thinking, research has established that natural levels of lactoferrin go up in response to viral infection. Folks at the National Institutes of Health in Bethesda, Maryland, examined the chemical makeup of nasal secretions (snot) to find out about lactoferrin levels [75]. In this research, sinuses of patients were exposed to rhinovirus type 39. Rhinovirus type 39 is a particular type of cold virus that has been genetically mapped out. They then rinsed out the sinuses of the participants (before and after viral exposure) and analyzed the rinse to get a better picture of what the body does in response to viral infection. The analysis of the nasal secretions showed that IgG, lactoferrin, lysozyme, and secretory IgA were increased after exposure. Does this list sound familiar? It's the same list of compounds that you find in colostrum. If the body increases its production of these compounds in response to a cold virus, it stands to reason that these same compounds are the virus busters for the body.

Lactoferrin has been shown to stop viral infections in their tracks [76]. When observed in a petri dish, both bovine lactoferrin and human lactoferrin inhibited the ability of a cold virus to reproduce itself in a dose-dependent manner. The more that lactoferrin was present in the petri dish, the greater the inhibition of the virus. On the basis of some additional findings in this study, these researchers concluded that most of the antiviral activity of lactoferrin takes place in the first phases of viral replication. So if you are thinking about taking colostrum for your next cold, you should consider starting yourself on the supplement as soon as possible when you are sick. I personally keep myself on a maintenance dose of colostrum so that it is always on board when my body is exposed to something bad. Similar findings have been found for lactoferrin and viral inhibition for human papillomavirus [77], hantavirus [78], and hepatitis B [79].

But how does lactoferrin stop viral infection? Colostrum doesn't need to destroy every single piece of virus to stop infection. All colostrum really has to do is slow down the spread of an invading virus long enough for the body to make enough antibodies to destroy it. (The same logic applies to how antibiotics work against bacteria.) Let's talk for a moment about how viruses infect cells. Essentially, a virus is a little piece of genetic code in a protein shell that cannot reproduce on its own. It wants to get inside your cells, take over the cells' genetic copying machinery, and use it to make more copies of itself. If a virus gets inside one of your cells, it can make thousands of copies of itself that then leave the cell and infect other cells. Each of your cells has a series of doors through which nutrients and other compounds are moved in and out. To get into a cell, the virus has to have a specific type of protein coat to get access to the door. Different viruses have different types of protein coats, and different cells have different types of doors. If the virus protein shell does not match the type of door on the cell, it cannot get in. That's why viruses that affect cells in your sinuses do not go on to infect your liver; the protein shell and the door do not match up.

In a study out of Japan, researchers attempted to determine which part of lactoferrin interacts with the hepatitis C virus and how lactoferrin prevents viral infection and proliferation. The study found that lactoferrin binds to the protein coat of the hepatitis virus [80]. Because the molecular shape of the virus protein coat is now changed, it cannot fit through the door of the liver cell. Because the virus cannot get inside to reproduce itself, it's very easy for the immune system to pounce on and destroy all existing copies. If we can get enough lactoferrin circulating in the body to bind to the protein coats of viruses, we can go a long way to preventing viral infection.

The complex formula that is colostrum has often been referred to as immune milk. Why? Because of its well understood and widely accepted benefits for the recipient's immune system.

But what about diseases that devastate the patient's immune system, such as HIV? Can colostrum offer any hope for AIDS patients? Thought leaders in immunology are now pointing toward colostrum for its ability to provide relief for the chronically HIV-infected patient [81]. It has even been suggested that the viral protein coat binding properties of colostrum may reduce the viral activity of HIV type 1 [74].

Colostrum defends the gut. One of the most potent properties of colostrum is its ability to heal the stomach and intestinal wall. Colostrum is particularly helpful for healing the digestive tract because all of the growth factors are readily available as it moves through the stomach into the colon, where it is absorbed. New research is suggesting that colostrum may be the next generation of treatment for poorly understood gastrointestinal disorders [82]. Colostrum is a hugely diverse and complex soup of compounds with a comparable diversity in its activity on the body. One compound in colostrum that influences the health of the gut is transforming growth factor α (TGF-α). This amino acid is produced naturally within the lining of the gastrointestinal tract [83]. Systemic administration of TGF-α triggers growth and cell repair of the stomach and intestines. It also reduces acid production and stimulates the mucosal lining of the gut to heal itself after injury [84]. Playford and his team [82] went on to say that the sheer complexity of the soup that is colostrum may be what causes it to be so effective on the body. In sum, this means that one peptide increases the activity of another and that multiple peptides increase the likelihood that the active compound will survive the stomach acid.

Playford and team [82] went on to list the many diverse gastrointestinal disorders for which colostrum could offer hope: short bowel syndrome, nonsteroidal anti-inflammatory drug-induced gut injury, chemotherapy-induced mucositis, inflammatory bowel disease, necrotizing enterocolitis, and infective diarrhea. Inflammatory bowel diseases, such as ulcerative colitis and Crohn's disease, are poorly understood and quite severe conditions for those who have them. Studies using an animal model of inflammatory bowel conditions and administration of the peptides found in colostrum (EGF, PDGF, TGF-β, or IGF-1) have provided encouraging results for the medical management of these conditions using colostrum. Significant improvement in inflammatory markers is very exciting. Clearly we need more human trials to determine colostrum dose requirements and to document cellular change. Colostrum may offer a novel way to manage these modern diseases.

Last, I wanted to tell you about some exciting research on healing gut damage that came about through the use of anti-inflammatory drugs. Our amazing friend colostrum is a health food supplement that prevents damage to the stomach and intestines from NSAIDs (nonsteroidal anti-inflammatory drugs). Many people rely on NSAIDs to manage pain and medical conditions from muscle injury to arthritis. By turning down the inflammation with a drug like ibuprofen, we reduce pain and allow the stressed muscle or tendon to heal. However, these drugs come with a considerable risk of damage to the lining of the stomach and intestines as a result of their use. In this study, the intestines of mice were injured with a compound called indomethacin [85]. (Poor little guys.) However, when the intestines of the mice were pretreated with colostrum, the gastric injury was reduced significantly. In fact, there was a dose-dependent effect such that mice with twice as much colostrum on board were twice as likely to be protected from damage.

Colostrum punches out cancer. Cancer is a devastating killer in today's world, responsible for 13 percent of all deaths globally, according to the World Health Organization [86]. Colostrum has been found to be active against various cancers, including Hodgkin's disease [87], osteogenic sarcoma [88], and prostate cancer [89]. To understand how colostrum works to protect us from cancer, let's talk about one way cancerous cells come about in the first place. As we age and die on the macro level, so, too, our individual cells age and die on the micro level. To replace the cells that die, the body has to make new ones. If you remember from your biology class, this process is called *cell division*. Every new cell needs a DNA road map to survive because our DNA governs all of the basic processes in our cells. For a cell to divide, the DNA has to be copied. When there are two copies of this DNA strand, the cell splits in two, with each new cell having a copy. Now, think about how many hundreds of thousands of DNA copies have been made since you were an infant—there are hundreds of thousands of opportunities for something to go wrong in the cell division process.

Think of cell division like a copy machine. The first time you make a paper copy, the copy looks practically identical to the original. However, there are tiny flaws in it—strands of hair, bent corners on the original, or dust on the glass can all cause imperfections in the copy. Now, make a copy of a copy, and even more errors are introduced into the final version. Once a flaw is introduced into your DNA, it has the potential to be passed along in all future divisions of the cell. Fortunately, there are repair enzymes that run up and down the DNA stand, checking for mutation errors like these and fixing them—kind of like white-out for the body. Still, DNA damage is considered to be one of the main agents in the aging process.

But how exactly can DNA copying errors cause cancer? Let's get even more technical. When genes are expressed, they make enzymes and chemical messengers that go to other parts of the cell to do work. Errors in DNA transcription can cause us to age prematurely. How does this work? Genes make proteins that turn into enzymes. These enzymes then govern DNA repair mechanisms. We could say that DNA manages itself because a piece of DNA makes an enzyme that turns around and checks it for errors. Through processes of oxidation, the building blocks of DNA called nucleotides (molecules made up of sugars and phosphate) can get fused together. When it is time to make this part of the DNA into a protein, an error occurs. The resulting protein is not made properly, and so it will not be able to do

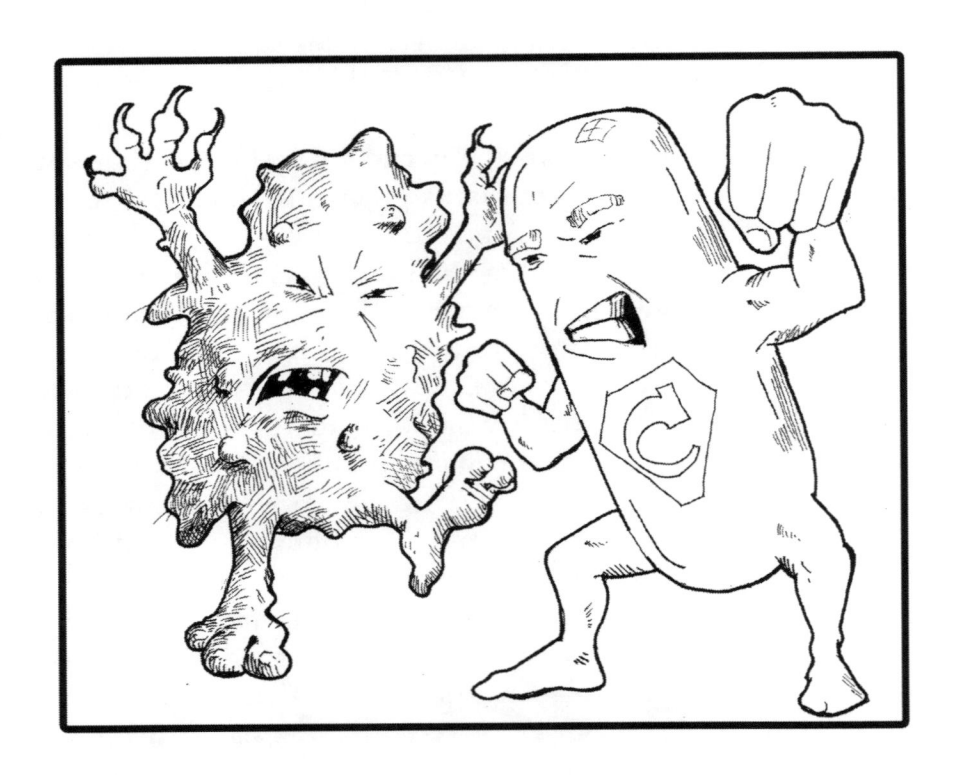

"Take that, you rogue."

its job as an enzyme. If this error occurs in a critical spot, the enzymes that are produced to control cellular regeneration can be flawed—resulting in cancerous overgrowth. To check for these fused nucleotides and correct them before they cause trouble, a different part of your DNA makes an enzyme that runs up and down the DNA strand, finding these fused nucleotides and breaking them apart. If fewer of these repair enzymes are coded for as we age because chemical messenger systems decline, then we run an increased cancer risk as we get older. The take-home message here is that DNA controls everything—especially aging.

In 2006, a study was published in the *Journal of Experimental Therapeutics and Oncology* that described the anticancer properties of PRP in colostrum [90]. Remember PRP from our discussion on immune modulation? The PRP in colostrum also reduces the frequency of spontaneous or induced DNA mutations, the root of cancer in the body. PRP in colostrum acts to assist your body's own DNA repair mechanisms and can reduce the frequency of DNA mutations in humans. An interesting and not well known fact about the human body is that cancer cells are forming *all* the time. Scary, I know. Your immune system is the only thing that diverts these cancerous cells from a total take-over. Your immune system is designed to seek out and destroy cancer cells before they have a chance to develop into malignant tumors. By enriching the body with immunoglobulins and protein-rich polypeptides from colostrum, you increase your ability to naturally repair your DNA and kill cancer cells. If the body doesn't detect and destroy cancer cells early, tumors will grow too big for the body to battle. As we age, the efficiency of these repair mechanisms declines, making us more vulnerable to errors in cell division as we age. Colostrum can help to return the body to a more youthful and efficient state of repair at the level of DNA.

Do you remember lactoferrin from our general discussion of the healing compounds in colostrum? It is an iron-binding protein that has a variety of physiological activities. Like PRP, lactoferrin has also been shown to inhibit carcinogenesis [91]. This magical protein suppresses the production of cancer cells in the human colon and in other organs of test animals [92]. In clinical trials, bovine lactoferrin was shown to reduce the risk of colon cancer in humans. In a review of immunohistochemical investigations conducted on cancer over the last twenty-five years, Tuccari and Barresi [93] concludes that lactoferrin is immune reactive and cancer suppressive in a variety of human tissue types. Lactoferrin acts as a chemical messenger and induces programmed cell death in cancer cells to inhibit their proliferation to other parts of the body [86]. Approximately fifty to seventy billion cells in your body die according to programmed cell death. But in the case of cancer, cells don't die when they are supposed to; they just keep reproducing and spreading. When lactoferrin enters the scene, it can differentiate cancer cells that are out of control through the innate chemicals that mark cancer cells. It then signals the cells to turn on their "death machinery," and the cells enter the same kind of programmed death that tells the cells between your fingers and toes to die when the human embryo is developing. How does it know? It's colostrum! And that means it's biochemical magic.

In Conclusion

In this chapter, I have introduced you to the anti-aging miracle that is colostrum. We talked about how epithelial repair factor and PRP help your skin step back from the brink of visible aging. We also discussed the general anti-aging properties of colostrum and how it can support your immune system. The benefits of colostrum are more than skin deep; they represent an alternative health model that can reinvent the way you live and care for your body. When people ask, "What's your secret?" just smile and tell them that you have been eating more carrots.

Chapter 5

The Master Menu

In this chapter, we discuss how to take colostrum and other nutritional supplements that are based on the science of its components. What should I look for in a colostrum product? What can I take if I am allergic to milk? What if I want to take a concentrated version of the active ingredients in colostrum? In this chapter, we review colostrum, monolaurin, IgG 2000 DF, and Viralox® Health Spray. Finally, we talk about detox reactions and what to expect when beginning on a program of immune support.

Colostrum

When I talk to people about the miracle of colostrum, I often get a few raised eyebrows. My sister's ex-boyfriend even thought that colostrum was something that came out of an animal's colon (*colostrum* sounds like *colon*) and that I was asking people to take a supplement made from animal feces. No! I am not asking you to have anything to do with feces or colons. If I can get people past the name *colostrum*, one of the next suspicions they raise is the problem of absorption. "Doesn't the stomach destroy the healing compounds in colostrum?" Fortunately, it does not. Remember, Mother Nature knows her stuff and has had hundreds of thousands of years to perfect a delivery system for colostrum. Consider how newborns in all mammal species get access to colostrum: they nurse with their mothers immediately after birth. The healing compounds of colostrum are absorbed through the stomach lining and digestive tract for all newborn mammals.

As hard evidence, researchers on the anti-inflammatory properties of human milk have shown that the anti-inflammatory agents in colostrum are resistant enough to survive digestive enzymes. That means that these compounds are expected to remain active in the gastrointestinal tract [94]. Do we have proof that oral supplementation with colostrum actually gets absorbed and makes it into the body where it can be used? In a study of athletes who were given oral colostrum, blood levels of IGF-1 and saliva levels of IgA were increased [61]. To the skeptics in the audience, rest assured that colostrum will get into your system from the digestive tract. Later in this chapter, we talk about some technologies that have been developed to increase the absorption of colostrum even more.

Taking colostrum will deliver repair growth factors wherever your body needs it most. Colostrum is available in many delivery systems, including powder, capsules, creams, and chewables. The type of delivery system you choose is determined by what impact you are trying to achieve by taking colostrum. Deciding how much to take and for how long is a very individual decision that you should make in consultation with your medical provider. If you simply want to use colostrum to repair a small section of the skin on your body, your face, for example, you may want to choose a colostrum cream and apply it as a cosmeceutical. Near the end of this book, we discuss how to turn your everyday moisturizer into a posh cosmeceutical by adding colostrum to it. This delivery system gets colostrum right where you need it, to the skin. However, you may want to use colostrum to repair the skin on your entire body or for its general immune- and performance-boosting effects. If you want to take colostrum as a supplement for its general health benefits, this is when consultation with your health provider comes into play. Think of this section as a way to get educated for your conversation with the doctor. Although colostrum is classified as a food, not as a drug, it has such a profound effect on the body that I recommend this conservative approach.

Colostrum is believed to be exceedingly safe where supplements are concerned. Keep in mind that all of the compounds in colostrum are produced naturally in your body. These compounds are already in your system, but by taking colostrum, you are simply increasing the bioavailability of compounds that your body already makes. Finally, colostrum is the first food for practically all the mammals on the planet. Mother Nature made this stuff to give newborns a fighting chance at survival. If Mother Nature gives colostrum to infants as their first food out of the womb, it stands to reason that it's pretty safe stuff.

Most people do not experience any side effects when taking bovine colostrum. Although most people do not experience side effects from colostrum, some patients who are HIV positive have anecdotally reported significant side effects such as abnormal liver function. So if you have a severely impaired immune system or are HIV positive, you should speak carefully with your doctor before beginning colostrum. You also should talk with your doctor about taking colostrum if you are pregnant or breast-feeding as the impact on the developing baby is unknown. Remember that pregnancy suppresses the immune system for a reason; any supplement that enhances the immune system could interfere with this natural suppressive effect and cause problems for the baby. Finally, you should avoid colostrum if you are allergic to cow's milk or milk products.

The big question on everyone's mind is how much colostrum to take when using it as an oral supplement. I personally take fifteen grams in the morning and fifteen grams in the afternoon to improve my skin, manage Lyme disease, and support my general health. Experts suggest that colostrum supplements should be taken in divided quantities, twice a day, because of the half-life rates of decay in the body. For example, a study looking at absorption of immunoglobulins for a group of newborn piglets indicated that the half-life of colostrum-derived antibodies in the bloodstream ranged from 3 to 17.7 days [95]. Whatever dose you choose, split it up between morning and evening. If I happen to have a cold or the flu, I even increase my amount in the short term.

What do the experts say about how much colostrum to take? Unless you are seeing a holistic physician with experience in recommending colostrum, your traditional provider may not know how much colostrum to recommend for you. Administration of colostrum should be conducted on an individual basis. Typical amounts start at one thousand milligrams of the powered form twice daily. By slowly increasing the amount you take, you can achieve the healing effect you desire.

In a review of colostrum research by the Institute of Colostrum Research [58], dosages of bovine (cow) colostrum in short-term, clinical studies ranged from twenty to sixty grams per day in powder form. This translates into 1.7 to 120 milligrams per day of the growth factor IGF-1. If you are thinking about supplementing your diet with colostrum to improve your athletic performance, colostrum is considered safe for this purpose. According to the Institute of Colostrum Research [58], there are no known contraindications to short-term supplementation with bovine colostrum for athletes. There are also no known precautions or warnings about the use of bovine colostrum for athletes. Finally, colostrum does not appear on the banned drug lists of the International Olympic Committee or any other sports governing bodies.

Experts have suggested different views about whether colostrum is safe to take if you are allergic to milk. On the conservative side, experts advise those who are milk intolerant to avoid colostrum. Conversely, a more liberal view observes that colostrum has very little lactose as compared to milk and may be perfectly safe. Although goat's colostrum can be purchased like bovine colostrum, most experts suggest that it is species specific and will do little to confer immunity to humans (only to other goats). However, there have been some anecdotal reports of benefit for humans from goat colostrum; you might consider experimenting with goat colostrum if you are allergic to milk. If you have problems with cow's milk, I would recommend that you consider one of the other supplements reviewed in this chapter that are based on the ingredients of colostrum. However, these other products will not contain the repair factors of colostrum that turn back the clock on skin. If you are using one of these other products for general health but would also like to address the visible signs of aging, consider using colostrum as a topical, as described later in this book.

What about colostrum for children? If you conduct a search on Amazon, you will find a plethora of chewable colostrum products for children. Short-term therapy of colostrum with children is considered generally safe. However, some thought leaders have cautioned against prolonged colostrum or lactoferrin-only therapy for children whose immune systems are still developing. Talk to your pediatrician about short-term colostrum therapy for when your child is sick. Remember, colostrum supplementation in adulthood is designed to counteract a decline in function of the immune system (the body makes less of the compounds the immune system uses as people age). Because children are not in this period of decline, it's unknown what effect immune-boosting compounds have on the feedback mechanisms of their developing immune systems.

The next question that people have about taking colostrum is which product to buy; there are many from which to choose. Doug Wyatt has charged the research arm of the Center for Nutritional Research to establish criteria for high-quality, bioavailable colostrum [96]. First, experts at the center say that the colostrum you purchase should have gone through pasteurization according to international standards; you don't want your colostrum to have pests. This process does not sterilize colostrum, but it does reduce the number of viable pathogens. Pasteurization should be conducted at 72 degrees Celsius for fifteen seconds and does not affect the bioavailability of the components. Aside from pasteurization, colostrum should be handled at low temperatures at all stages of preparing it for market. As soon as it is collected, the colostrum you buy should be kept cool. If it is exposed to heat for too long, the immune proteins will become denatured and break down. Third, colostrum that you purchase should clearly state values for its components, including IGF, immunoglobulins, lactoferrin, and EGF. A high-quality product will provide values for multiple immunoglobulins, including IgG, IgM, and IgA.

Unfortunately at this time, there is no international standard for how much immunoglobulin and lactoferrin colostrum should contain. If the manufacturer uses additives, make sure these additives are inert (not enzymes, for example) with no capacity to break down the active ingredients in colostrum. Your colostrum should be collected after the newborn calf has nursed for its needs and within twelve hours of birth. Finally, some producers of colostrum have attempted to increase the stability of colostrum by shielding it from the stomach acid with a protective coating. Experts believe that adding this type of coating to a colostrum product will increase its absorbability by up to eight times. One example of this processing technology is a liposomal delivery system, or Colostrum-LD by Sovereign Laboratories. This delivery system coats the colostrum in the same lipids that make up cell membranes, affording it protection from stomach acids. Another producer of colostrum uses a protective enzyme called chymosin to guard colostrum from stomach acid. Regardless, check the label on the product you buy and look for a product that uses a delivery technology that protects the colostrum from stomach acid.

MONOLAURIN

The next supplement that we discuss is called monolaurin. Monolaurin is a compound in breast milk that has been shown to have bacteriocidal and fungicidal properties. Today, monolaurin is isolated from coconut oil and made available for purchase as a nutritional supplement. Using an electron microscope to determine its mechanism of action, monolaurin was shown to break apart biological membranes and cell walls of bacteria and fungi [97,98]. Thus monolaurin has demonstrated activity against bacteria, including *E. coli,* staph, and *Bacillus subtilis,* while activity has been demonstrated against fungi, including *C. albicans, Aspergillus niger,* and *Penicillium expansum.* Monolaurin also has potential as a broad-spectrum antibacterial agent when applied topically for either animals or humans [99]. Monolaurin is the most effectively used under the guidance of your health care provider.

IgG 2000 DF

Of course, if you are allergic to milk, colostrum may not be the best choice for you. If you happen to be in this boat, the supplement community has begun formulating nutritional supplements that provide isolated ingredients from colostrum, such as lactoferrin, immunoglobulins, and cysteine. These supplements may be of possible benefit for those milk-intolerant people who really need the general health-boosting effects of colostrum. Unfortunately, these products do not appear to contain the growth factors found in natural colostrum and so are unlikely to improve the health and appearance of your skin.

One product, called IgG 2000 DF, by Xymogen, is a revolutionary new proprietary formulation of some of the best ingredients of colostrum. Offered in capsule or powder form, this supplement provides a broad spectrum of immunoglobulins, including IgG, IgA, IgM, IgE, and IgD. This nondairy source of immunoglobulins boasts three times the amount of IgG found in colostrum. It also delivers fifteen times the amount of lactoferrin than colostrum for aggressive immune support. This supplement is particularly helpful in maintaining a healthy balance of friendly intestinal bacteria as it delivers immune support factors right to the digestive tract. Get yourself cleared by your doctor on this supplement for general immune support or for digestive concerns such as food poisoning, bacterial imbalance, or candida overgrowth.

Laura Flynn Geissel, PhD

VIRALOX® HEALTH SPRAY

In chapter 4, we discussed two very important components of colostrum: PRP and lactoferrin. I also shared clinical research using a PRP spray with HIV/AIDS patients to decrease viral counts, decrease malaise, and increase the activity of CD4+ lymphocytes [56]. The oral spray used in this research is now available for individual purchase and combines some of the best components of colostrum in a novel delivery system. Viralox® Health Spray by Sovereign Laboratories helps rebuild and rebalance the immune system. Although individual results may vary, supplementation with this oral spray can help reduce the inflammatory response while increasing the pathogen-destroying power of the immune system. The lactoferrin in this spray attaches itself to viruses, preventing them from entering cells and spreading throughout the body. Evidence suggests that the general immune-building effects of this spray also make it effective against nonviral pathogens such as bacteria and fungi. Initial findings suggest that the cellular messengers in Viralox® can increase the killing power of our own natural killer cells by up to 200 percent, even in people with compromised immune systems.

A WORD ON DETOX REACTIONS

All of the literature you will read on colostrum will tell you that colostrum is a food, not a medication. But in my opinion, the healing impact of colostrum goes far beyond what we can expect from ordinary food. For example, a carrot provides essential nutrients, but it does not provide the body with the basic building blocks of the immune system. When taking colostrum, it is important to begin slowly and build up to the quantity that gives you the healing effect you desire. You don't have to build up slowly on other foods, but this is the best practice that I recommend for maximizing your outcome with this supplement.

Bovine colostrum is considered by all the authors that I reviewed for this book to be generally safe. In some cases, people who have taken colostrum have reported mild flulike symptoms that remitted with continued use of the supplement. This reaction is called *detox* by the naturopathic community. I want to describe the detox reaction in more detail because any person may experience detox when first starting on any of the supplements that I review in this chapter. If something supercharges your immune system, a detox reaction can happen at the beginning of therapy.

Detox may feel bad for a while, but it is actually a good thing. Detox basically means that your body is fighting harder to rid itself of subclinical infections. Today, the naturopathic community recognizes a number of mild detox reactions or "healing crises." However, the very first type of detox reaction was documented in 1895 by the traditional medical community; it was called the Jarisch–Herxheimer reaction. Adolf Jarisch and Karl Herxheimer are credited with the discovery of this reaction when they were working with patients being treated with mercury for syphilis. Back then, doctors did not have antibiotics, and so mercury was used to treat life-threatening infections. This reaction is also well understood in modern times as being a reaction to the first administration of antibiotics for syphilis and tick-borne illnesses. Symptoms can develop within the first few hours of antibiotic administration, including fever, chills, rigor, hypotension, headache, racing heartbeat, hyperventilation, flushing, muscle pain, and anxiety. What causes this type of reaction? When the antibiotic begins to kill off the invading organisms, endotoxins and lipoproteins are dumped into the body faster than it can remove them. As these compounds build up over a matter of hours, the symptoms of the Jarisch–Herxheimer reaction develop. Fortunately, these types of reactions are self-limiting, as the body is able to remove more of the offending compounds over time. They can also remit with the administration of an anti-inflammatory drug.

Even if you do not carry a diagnosis of syphilis or a tick-borne illness, you can experience a mild form of the Jarisch-Herxheimer reaction when beginning on an immune-boosting supplement like colostrum. How does this work? According to the naturopathic community, we all carry subclinical levels of invasive pathogens in our bodies. Maybe you don't believe that the body carries subclinical infections. But in fact, bacteria outnumber our cells by ten to one. Many of these bacteria are unfriendly organisms that are simply waiting for an opportunity when the body's defenses lapse. This means that the body is constantly engaged in defending itself and keeping these invaders at low levels. Your immune system is working constantly to manage your unique and individual load of bacterial, viral, and fungal residents. Think of your body like a piece of bread that you left out on the table for too long — within a couple of days, mold spores that have fallen on the bread have totally taken over. Without the immune system's constant work, your body would look like this piece of bread in a short time. I even had one holistic doctor tell me that our subclinical load of fungi increases as we age to prepare for death, when fungi will be needed to decompose our physical being. Thanks, Doc, but I'm not ready yet.

One example of a subclinical infection is invasive yeast, a type of fungi. With the increasing use of antibiotics over the lifetime, an individual can deplete the beneficial bacteria that help to keep invasive fungi from spreading. Think of the tissues in your body like an apartment building. If the good bacteria are renting all of the apartments, then there is less of a chance that invasive fungi can move into the building. Basically, good bacteria take up the space, blocking invading yeasts from moving in. If the good bacteria get depleted from repeated antibiotic use, then invasive yeast (candida) can move into the empty spaces and cause lots of problems.

Let's go forward with the hypothesis that most of us have had more than one round of antibiotics in our lifetime and so carry more invasive yeast than we should. Imagine that we have one million yeast organisms in the digestive tract that should not be there. Now, along comes colostrum, which you just took as an oral supplement. Colostrum delivers lactoferrin and immunoglobulins directly to your digestive tract. There is an excellent chance that the cow who produced your colostrum was also exposed to invasive fungi and yeasts. (Fungi are everywhere!) That cow would have developed immunoglobulins specific for yeast to be passed on to its offspring. By taking colostrum, you receive passive immunity for any organism to which the cow was exposed. So, you just took a big dose of immunoglobulins specific for invasive yeast. What happens now? Your body shifts into a hyperdrive immune response to destroy invasive yeast with the new defensive weapons it just received from colostrum. In a matter of a few days, you might kill off half a million yeast organisms. Endotoxins and lipoproteins from the dead yeast are dumped into the digestive tract and absorbed into the bloodstream. Because of this rapid die-off, there are more endotoxins than the body can effectively process. These elevated levels cause a mild version of a Jarisch–Herxheimer reaction that can include flulike symptoms, headache, mild fever, body aches, increased mucus production, and so on. Over time, the body catches up as the death of invading organisms tapers off and the symptoms of detox naturally remit.

As a person with Lyme disease, detox reactions are part of my everyday life. When I was going through aggressive antibiotic therapy, the detox when I first began antibiotics was so severe that I was off work for a week with fever, body aches, joint swelling, headache, dizziness, insomnia, and anxiety attacks. Unfortunately, the toxins from Lyme affect multiple body systems, and detox symptoms can include muscular and skeletal problems, neurological problems, and general malaise. Currently I am not taking any antibiotics for Lyme. However, the same antibiotics that are prescribed for sinus problems also kill Lyme. I dread having to take antibiotics for sinus infections because I then go through all of the Lyme detox symptoms in addition to being sick from sinus problems. It's really a challenge. Now that I am no longer taking antibiotics for Lyme, I am on a constant search for what concoction of nutritional herbs and supplements will help me to remain healthy. I know when I have happened on something that works for killing Lyme because I go through mild detox as an indicator. I take herbs for Lyme that have this effect. However, I have also noticed detox reactions whenever I add a new, immune-boosting supplement like colostrum. If you have a diagnosable clinical infection, like Lyme, or a nondiagnosable subclinical infection, you could experience mild detox symptoms from beginning colostrum too quickly.

Herxheimer-like reactions, including flulike symptoms, can occur at the beginning of therapy for some generally healthy people who take colostrum. These symptoms are part of the healing process; they are usually mild and disappear with continued use of the same amount of colostrum. To avoid detox reactions, the best approach is to start out with a small amount of one thousand milligrams of colostrum twice a day. If, after five days, you are not experiencing any detox symptoms, up your daily intake by one thousand milligrams. Continue increasing your quantity every five days until you reach the desired healing effect. If you experience mild detox reactions, you can go back down to the previous level for a longer period of time. Anecdotally, some people take sixty grams a day of colostrum to achieve specific healing goals; the amount a person takes is very individual. Remember, when you take one of these healing foods, you should be working with your doctor closely regarding any significant detox reactions. Finally, if you have a significant medical condition and your doctor has told you that it is OK to begin one of these compounds, you may want to increase your dose even more slowly. Slow and steady wins the race.

Chapter 6

Understanding Inflammation (and Why You Should Care)

What Is Inflammation?

INFLAMMATION IS ONE OF THE main harbingers of the aging process. When the body activates chronic inflammatory procedures, it sets in motion a series of biochemical processes that interfere with proper function of the body. An easy way to understand inflammation is to think about what happens when you get a piece of dust in your eye. How does the eye respond? It gets red as blood rushes to the area, puffy, and perhaps tearful to wash out the invading dust. All of these symptoms are signs of inflammation. Inflammation is the body's response to protect and heal itself. If the dust is removed, the body returns to its healthy, uninflamed state. But if you keep putting dust in the eye, it stays in a chronically inflamed state. Over time, the eye will develop chronic problems from too many inflammatory symptoms.

Inflammation can be categorized as either acute or chronic. Another easy example of acute inflammation is a cut in the skin. What happens during acute inflammation? When you cut yourself, the cut becomes red and puffy as blood and repair mechanisms rush to the area to heal the break in the skin [100]. Inflammation brings healing factors to the area and the cut heals.

When the body responds to a harmful invader (like bacteria, fungi, or viruses), it responds by initially moving plasma and leukocytes from the blood to the tissue that is being affected. This process usually wraps up in a few hours to a few days and is characterized by five signs: pain, redness, immobility or loss of function, swelling, and heat. If you think back to a recent muscle injury, you should be able to remember all of these telltale signs of inflammation. Inflammation in response to a respiratory virus can also be described by these classic signs: pain (sinus pressure or headache), redness (red nose or cheeks), loss of function (inability to smell), swelling (puffy cheeks or nose), and heat (fever).

The body is designed to operate using acute inflammation to solve its problems. The crucial factor is that the inflammation resolves and goes away in a normal healthy response. Problems happen for the body when inflammation becomes chronic and does not resolve. This chronic inflammation can last for years and can be caused by (1) inability to eliminate whatever was causing the acute inflammation; (2) the immune system mistaking healthy tissue for a foreign invader, as in autoimmune disorders; and (3) a chronic invader of a subclinical nature that the body just can't get rid of. Unfortunately, a fourth source of inflammation is inflammation itself. Inflammation can cause more inflammation and become self-perpetuating. Some examples of diseases that develop through chronic inflammation include coronary artery disease, rheumatoid arthritis, and psoriasis. Other problems believed to have an inflammatory component include asthma, celiac disease, inflammatory bowel disease, skin aging, transplant rejection, and acne.

Immune activation and inflammation are like two sides of the same coin. If we can enhance the effectiveness of the immune system, the body will need less inflammation to clear an invader. Less inflammation means there is less stuff for your body to clean up after an insult as it returns to normal. For example, your nose runs (inflammation) for days, even after the infection has cleared, because inflammatory processes have been turned on. When the cold is gone, the body needs to use further actions from the immune system to bring down the inflammation in the nose such as stopping mucus production and reducing swollen tissues. What if we could teach your nose to stop running at the exact time that the infection has been eradicated? Furthermore, if we can clear infection while reducing the amount of inflammation that the body uses to do it, then less healing needs to take place after a traumatic event. If the immune system is freed up from healing the sequlae of inflammation, then it is free to do other work, like preventing infection or attacking cancer cells before they get a chance to reproduce.

Finally, chronic inflammatory processes can reduce the ability of the immune system to do its job. Researchers in the Immunonutrition Research Group out of Spain have discussed obesity as a condition in which the immune system is compromised through inflammatory confusion [101]. In their research, they observed that inflammatory processes associated with obesity explain obesity-related immune deficiency. They relate the increase of pro-inflammatory compounds (leptin) and a decrease in anti-inflammatory compounds (adiponectin) to the decreased activation of immune cells. This is why inflammation is important and why you should care; it reduces the effectiveness of your immune system. Think of it like a battle. The worst thing that can happen in battle is to get surrounded on all sides by the enemy. You can't fight nine guys at once; at best, you can only deal with one or two. If your immune system is busy battling its own tissue, it has reduced resources to use when battling an actual enemy.

Chronic inflammation either means that the immune system is confused and working on the wrong problem or that there is a persistent invader that is beyond your internal resources to manage. Either way, the goal in anti-aging science is to limit and heal inflammation. Now we are going to talk about diet as a primary strategy for limiting inflammation and therefore freeing up your immune system to work on actual problems.

Laura Flynn Geissel, PhD

DIET AND INFLAMMATION

"You are what you eat" is an old saying. In fact, it turns out to be true. As we begin our discussion of inflammation, we will first talk about poor skin health as a way of understanding this concept. A very comprehensive study was conducted in 2001 by researchers from Monash University, Melbourne, Australia, about what types of food contribute to healthy skin [102]. They also investigated what types of food are related to poor skin health. Good-for-you, anti-inflammatory diets (veggies, fruit, nonprocessed foods, nuts, fish, and low sugar) were related to a lack of wrinkles in the people studied. If you want to use diet to help reduce overall levels of inflammation, the following foods are recommended:

- Olive oil and olives
- Fish high in essential fatty acids such as sardines and salmon
- Eggs
- Legumes such as peas, chickpeas, broad beans, and lima beans
- Foods high in vitamin C, such as peaches, citrus fruits, and fruit juices
- Vegetables, such as spinach, eggplant, celery, leeks, garlic, and onions
- Carotenoid-rich fruits and vegetables (cantaloupe, apricots, carrots, and sweet potatoes)
- Avocados
- All types of berries
- Whole-grain cereals
- All fruits and fruit juices
- Foods high in zinc, such as seafood, nuts, milk, and lean meats

Water and tea

On the flip side, following are the foods you should avoid to slow down the aging and inflammatory processes of your skin:

Saturated fats

Red meat and processed meats

Full-fat dairy products

Carbonated drinks

Alcohol

Refined sugar

Candies and sweets

White flour

Potatoes

Margarine

So, we now know that an anti-inflammatory diet, filled with fresh items like fruits, vegetables, and whole, unprocessed foods, can help you keep inflammation to a minimum over time. One rule of thumb here is that any food that does not get to you in its own natural package is likely to contribute to inflammation. As you looked over the list of anti-inflammatory foods, you were probably thinking, "Man, this is going to be work!" And you were right—anti-inflammatory foods are not as readily available in our fast-food and highly processed food culture. When we think about eating a cheeseburger versus a fresh salad, most of us feel more desire for the inflammatory cheeseburger meal (including beef, white flour bun, fried potatoes, and lots of fat). I often find myself lamenting inside, "Why do my desires and taste buds betray me? I want to love salad, not croissants!"

Why do our taste buds betray us? Why do we crave French fries and ice cream instead of salad? In this volume, scientific reasoning based in the theory of evolution forms the basis for the arguments presented about the origins of good health. Let's go back about a half million years, when human beings were just being formed. At this time, evolution was in full swing, selecting for adaptive genetics. The human beings you see today are the result of a series of genetic selections by a hostile and unforgiving environment. (However, I have never understood the great split between creationism and Darwinism. Isn't natural selection God's way of getting there?)

Let's consider the diet of a prehuman hundreds of thousands of years ago. See any fast food anywhere? Ice cream? Frozen dinners? No, you won't find any of these things. What you will find is what we now refer to as the anti-inflammatory, whole food diet. The main point here is that the food menu on which our digestive, immune, and cardiac systems developed is very different than it is today. Prehumans were eating mostly plants, with the occasional bit of meat or fish, when it could be caught. Also remember that there was no grocery store when the digestive system developed; it was very difficult to eat meat three times a day, like we often do now. Because what were available were mostly plants and small amounts of meat, prehumans who handled these foods more effectively were more likely to survive and pass on their genetics than those who did not. Genetically speaking, our bodies were engineered by the environment (with God directing behind the curtain, if you prefer) to perform well on the anti-inflammatory diet. Take that preperson away from that diet, and you take her away from good health.

The bodies in which we live were not designed to function on the highly processed fast-food menu on which we subsist today. Imagine that you bought a high-performance sports car. And when you bought it, the saleswoman told you to fill it only with high-octane fuel. Would you then go to the gas station and fill it with regular because it was a little bit cheaper? No, you would never treat your sports car that way. If you were to fill it with regular, you would experience a reduction in performance and could perhaps damage the engine over time. You would be crazy to fill it with regular after investing all that money in the car. But that is what we do with our diets every day. We seem to take better care of our things than we do of ourselves.

It would seem that we are wired to crave the things that are bad for us. Imagine our prehuman friend sitting on a rock somewhere in Africa. What is he craving? Actually, he is craving the same thing that you are craving: sugar and fat. Remember, Mother Nature selected us to have these cravings. Those prehumans who craved sugar and fat were more likely to survive and pass on their sugar and fat craving genetics into the pool of prehumans. Why did these prepeople survive? The only way to get sugar in prehistoric times was to eat fruit. Sugar-seeking fruit eaters were more likely to obtain essential vitamins (like vitamin C) than non-sugar-seeking prepersons. Thus sugar seekers survived and thrived to pass along their genetics to their offspring. We can extrapolate a similar mechanism for those who craved fat. Those whose taste buds told the brain to crave fat were more likely to seek out meat-filled diets. These fat seekers were more likely to obtain needed protein and store calories in the form of fat for lean times when food was less available. So when the occasional famine hit, the fat seeker had stored up enough calories to survive to better times. You can see now how your body is wired to go after sugar and fat—two core components of an inflammatory diet.

The modern problem is in the amount of fat and sugar ingested. In today's world, our main source of sugar is not fruit. Our cravings for sugar can lead us to consume a cup or more of raw sugar a day. In prehistoric times, there were limits on how much sugar and fat could be consumed because these items were not readily available. So not only are we eating excessive amounts of sugar today but our sugar sources are not providing us with important vitamins and minerals. The easy availability of sugar and fat in today's world has led us to the multiple health crises of obesity, heart disease, and many other conditions that can be tracked back to poor nutrition.

When we think about natural selection, we first think about something that happened a long time ago. But the truth of the matter is that natural selection is happening right now. Our

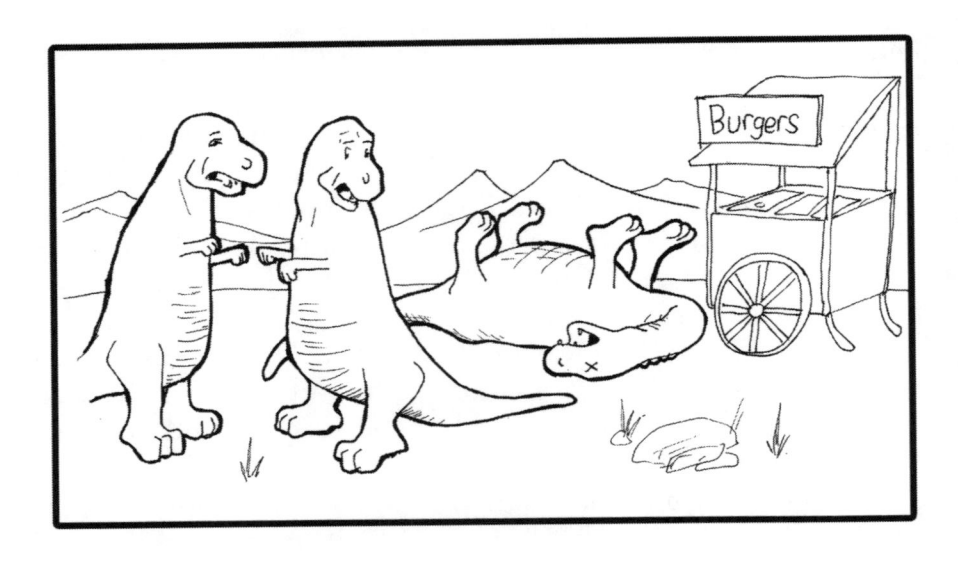

The real reason for the demise of the dinosaurs.

culture has experienced a cataclysmic change in diet. Those people who develop food-related health problems are being selected against by our fast-food environment. Perhaps in fifty thousand years or so, natural selection will have run its course and the human population that survives will be able to thrive on a highly processed food menu. But for now, our best option is to return our bodies to the dietary conditions under which they were designed to function.

Let's talk more about the prehistoric diet so that we can really understand what inflammation is, why it is bad, and what we can do to prevent it. What happens in the body when we ask it to process a food for which it is not designed? Simply put, the body responds to the food like it is an invader and marshals a defense. You will recognize this reaction as inflammation from our previous discussion. This model for inflammation happens throughout the body when we eat a diet high in processed foods, sugar, and fat. Chronic exposure to a dietary irritant is a major contributor to chronic inflammation that can spread out from the digestive tract and affect other organs in the body.

Because our digestive systems were not designed to digest processed food, the immune factors in the digestive tract respond like the food is an invader, marshaling a defense in the form of inflammation. Another example of a dietary irritant is a genetically modified organism (GMO) that is consumed as food. We can react to the altered proteins in genetically modified foods and marshal an allergic, inflammatory response. A GMO is any plant, animal, bacterium, insect, or fungus that has had its genetic material altered by science using techniques from genetic engineering. In genetic engineering, the DNA of the organism is altered, usually by inserting or removing specific genes. This can be accomplished by using a virus to deliver genetic material to the host organism or by manually inserting the new DNA with a syringe or gene gun [103]. The modified organism then passes its new genetic material on to its offspring, and an entirely new living entity is born. Examples of GMOs that science has recently created include bacteria that make insulin for diabetics [104], super fish [105], and fluorescent pigs [106].

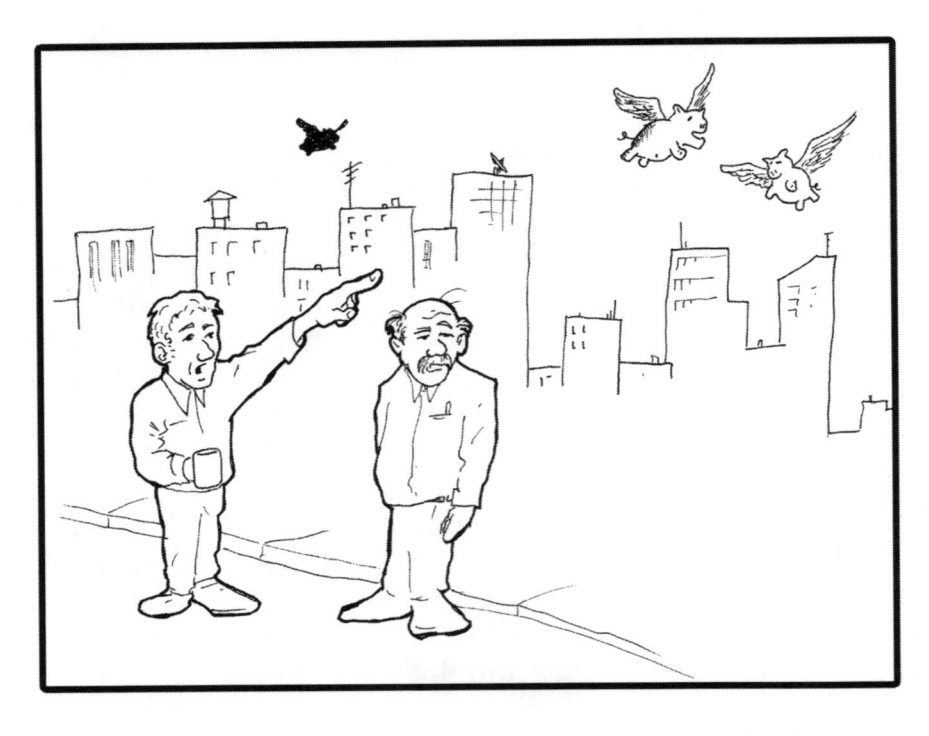

"There goes the newest GMO. Guess pigs do fly."

The Youth Prescription

You may be thinking, who needs a fluorescent pig? But actually these animals are used in some very targeted medical research.

When it comes to GMOs, there are two sides to the debate. On one side are proponents of research to discover and create new living things through genetic manipulation. These folks cite all the medical advances we now have because of medical research conducted with genetically modified plants, animals, and bacteria. If you happen to be a diabetic who depends on insulin produced by genetically modified bacteria, then you have a lot of gratitude for GMOs. Also, proponents of GMOs also talk about our greater ability to feed the world with genetically enhanced livestock, fish, and plants. It is hard to argue with the very real and tangible benefits that we have gained from GMOs.

However, I would like to argue that GMOs are a Pandora's box that we will never get shut again. Organisms with new genetic code are being released into the environment at an alarming and increasing rate. Changes in genetic code that used to require thousands of years in historical evolutionary processes are now being executed by scientists in a matter of months. I have a hard time with the idea that the limited scope of human awareness is a good substitute for the wisdom of Mother Nature. Nature uses a process of gradual trial and error to test out new genetic code. But GMOs are now impacting the fragile balance of plants, animals, and bacteria in ways that we don't know and can't predict.

As a model for how GMOs can impact our environment, think about what happens when a new species of plant or animal is brought into an area of the world where it doesn't belong. For example, a marine algae from the Mediterranean Sea, called *Caulerpa taxifolia,* was introduced in 2000 to the waterways and wetlands of California. Thought to be introduced by dumping the contents of household aquariums into storm drains, this algae forms a thick underwater blanket that kills other underwater vegetation. The resident birds and fish have no use for the algae, and so it grows unchecked and is unusable in the new environment. GMOs have the potential to impact our environment just like these marine species. When they enter the ecosystem, they may be so different from resident plants and animals that they disrupt the fragile ecological balance. But at least with our invasive species example, it's something from planet Earth that nature made! We have no idea how test-tube organisms will affect our ecosystem when they are either purposefully released or escape. Does Dr. Frankenstein ring any bells here? I sure hear them!

You may be wondering whether there is any evidence to suggest that an inflammatory diet actually causes inflammation that science can measure. I'm glad you asked, because there are scientific data to support this claim. Ingesting food that is high in saturated fat and high in calories has been correlated with an increase in inflammatory markers [107]. The authors suggest that even though the inflammatory response was acute in response to overeating, it could become chronic if the overeating is chronic. If we can keep on an anti-inflammatory diet, we can help prevent the immune system from becoming confused to the point of attacking things it should leave alone. We also discussed how processed foods can be interpreted as allergens, causing inflammation of the digestive tract. Signs of this type of inflammation include acid reflux, constipation, diarrhea, bloating, and gas. Like with processed foods, the human digestive tract was not exposed to GMOs when it developed. I want you to consider the possibility that a diet high in GMOs can begin the same cycle of chronic inflammation we see for processed foods. In sum, stick with the foods nature spent thousands of years developing and that come in natural packages.

The Anti-inflammatory Meal Replacement Smoothie

If you are a busy person like I am, it is just hard to get five to seven servings of fruits and vegetables a day. When I'm having a super busy day, I'm embarrassed to say that I look back over my day and see that I only had one serving. If you are like me, it can sometimes be unrealistic to spend forty minutes preparing and eating a salad. I had to find a quick and easy way to up my consumption of fruits and vegetables. The following recipe is based on the idea that you can eat anything if it has enough chocolate in it. I found a way to get down five servings of fruits and vegetables with about five minutes of prep time. Forget about bottled smoothies or weight loss drinks; this is the only meal replacement you will need. Replace lunch or dinner with a great meal that heals the body and reduces inflammation.

Another plus about this shake is that it delivers raw anti-inflammatory ingredients. When we cook our food, the heat destroys many of the naturally occurring enzymes and vitamins that your body needs. At the same time, I just do not believe in the raw-food diet. Cooking also releases soluble fiber and makes certain other vitamins more available. You need to manage your nutrition like your stock portfolio: diversify. Eat a mix of some cooked and some raw foods. For most of us, we tend to focus on a diet filled with cooked foods. That's where this shake comes in as an easy way to balance your diet with raw items.

Let's look at each ingredient in the shake and why it is good for you.

Ingredient	Nutritional value	Benefits
8 oz. of raw spinach	2 g protein 1.5 g of fiber	A green superfood that is a great source of iron, vitamin C, B vitamins, and vitamin E
2 medium carrots	1 g protein 4 g of fiber	A wonderful source of vitamin A and vitamin C
1 frozen banana	1.5 g protein 3 g of fiber	A great source of a hard-to-find mineral, potassium; the saying "an apple a day keeps the doctor away" really should be revised for the banana.
1 cup frozen cherries	1.5 g protein 3 g of fiber	A powerful anti-inflammatory, this berry has lately been proposed as a major preventive for gout and other types of arthritic inflammation
1 cup rice milk	Using the fortified brand provides additional vitamins	Adds a creamy taste to the smoothie without adding the inflammatory properties of milk

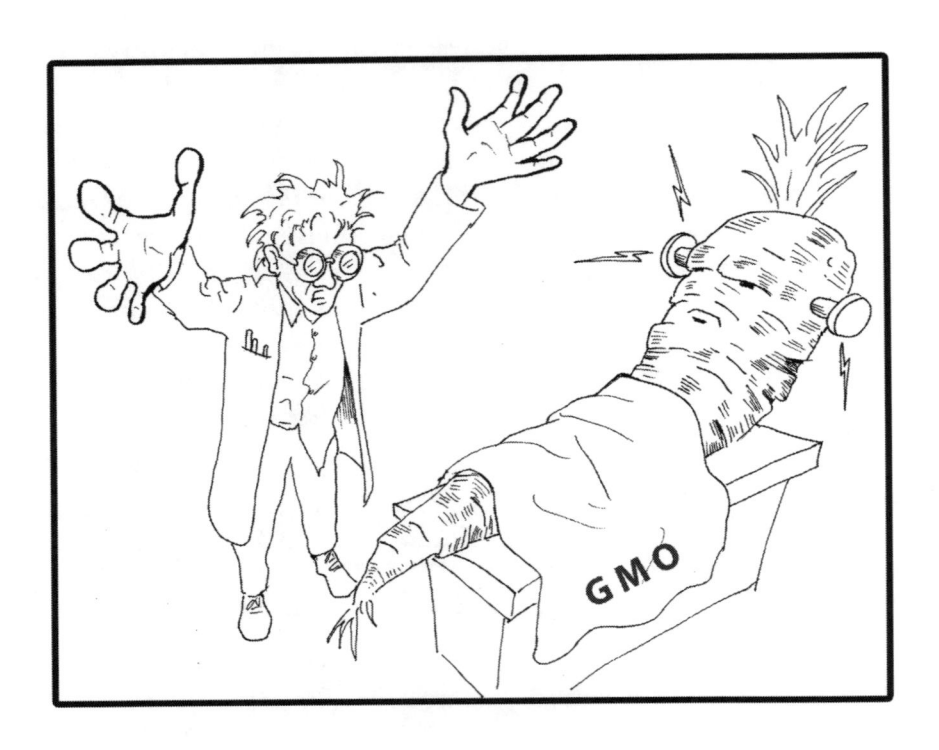

"Rise!"

1-4 tablespoons unsweetened cocoa powder		Lowers risk of heart disease; improves blood flow and circulation
1 scoop soy protein powder	18 g protein	Make this smoothie last like a meal and helps prevent the return of hunger
Ice cubes		Hydrates the body and numbs the taste buds to help get those veggies down

Put the preceding ingredients in the blender and process for three to five minutes. If the final smoothie is too thick for you, reduce by one carrot. Drink it within the first ten minutes, as the ingredients will start to separate over time. If you are allergic to chocolate, consider adding decaffeinated instant coffee crystals to cover over the flavor of the veggies. You can also consider a roasted coffee substitute like Pero for flavor variety.

INFLAMMATION AND THE MASTER ANTI-AGING SUPPLEMENT

We spent an entire chapter discussing why colostrum is the master anti-aging supplement. So, can colostrum be a Superman to the Lex Luther of chronic inflammation? Rock on, Superman. Bovine colostrum has been shown to be a powerful anti-inflammatory for the body. Researchers have tried to get a close approximation of the human response to colostrum while using an animal model. These folks actually used colostrum from human mothers and injected it into mice that were exposed to an inflammatory agent [108]. This was one of the first studies to demonstrate a measurable reduction in inflammatory markers in response to human colostrum. Many other studies since have demonstrated further evidence for the anti-inflammatory properties of colostrum [109].

A fire extinguisher for the body. Colostrum is a complex nutritional soup of healing compounds. In fact, the complexity of its makeup has been a challenge for scientists who were trying to figure out what the active ingredients are in the soup that contribute so magnificently to human health. One of the main compounds, lactoferrin, has received a great deal of attention by the scientific community. Lactoferrin, a component of colostrum, has been thoroughly researched as an anti-inflammatory agent. When the body is exposed to an irritant or invader, it increases production of its own lactoferrin. Lactoferrin production is increased during airway inflammation [110], gut inflammation [111], and when exposed to allergens. In other words, when the body is trying to solve its own inflammatory problems that cause inflammation, lactoferrin is the compound it mobilizes. By extension, we can increase the body's ability to clear inflammation by giving it more of this compound. Enter colostrum. When the body is under stress, you can either wait for it to produce its own lactoferrin, or you can help it out by adding colostrum to your system.

Colostrum heals inflammatory skin conditions. When skin is inflamed, it just doesn't look good. It may look red and puffy with visible capillaries and enlarged pores. Definitely not a good look on anyone. To get beautiful skin, we need to take down the inflammation and keep it down. Evidence about the link between skin aging and inflammation continues to mount. This link began to be described twenty-five years ago by Lavker and Kligman [112], who observed the impact of inflammation on the skin at the microscopic level. By some experts, cellular inflammation is considered to be the underlying factor in aging of the skin. Not only does skin aging get accelerated by external factors such as UV radiation but internal factors like inflammation also great a huge role in dictating the aging processes of the skin.

Most undesirable skin conditions can be linked to too much inflammation. Fortunately, the lactoferrin in colostrum can make an overactive immune system more moderate in the skin [113]. It does this by inhibiting local production of a compound called cytokine. To investigate the role of lactoferrin in reducing skin inflammation, researchers applied a topical allergen to the skin of mice and observed a dose-dependent inhibition of inflammation by lactoferrin [114]. (*Dose-dependent* means that the more lactoferrin that was administered to the skin, the greater the anti-inflammatory effect was seen to be.) Because lactoferrin is a compound that is produced normally in the skin [114,115], it makes sense that supplementing the skin's own anti-inflammatory mechanism with exogenous lactoferrin would lead to a dose-dependent reduction in skin inflammation.

Yet, do these findings about lactoferrin and inflammation extend beyond an animal model to humans? Actually, they do. (But you had that figured out already, right?) Researchers used human volunteers and treated their skin with a contact allergen (diphencyprone) in the presence and absence of topically applied lactoferrin [116]. Skin biopsies of the volunteers were then taken and evaluated. Exposure to the allergen was associated with an increase in inflammatory markers (erythema and leukocytes), whereas exposure to lactoferrin was associated with a decrease in these same skin inflammatory markers. Basically, this research documents that topical applications of a lactoferrin-containing compound, such as bovine colostrum, can give skin a real boost in its anti-inflammatory properties. We can also assume that this effect at the skin level can be extended throughout the body when we take a lactoferrin-containing supplement like colostrum.

Acne vulgaris is an inflammatory disease of the skin that involves a self-perpetuating process of inflammation. Having healthy skin isn't just about preventing and healing wrinkles; it's also about bolstering the skin against attack by the environment. In the case of acne, invasive bacteria become trapped in a pore of the skin, where they multiply into a local infection. The body responds to the infection with inflammation: blood (including white blood cells and other agents the body uses to fight infection) rushes to the infected area and battles the unfriendly bacteria. Dead bacteria (in the form of white pus) are pushed out of the pore to the surface of the skin by lymph fluid that has accumulated in the area. Regrettably, increased blood flow and immune factors don't just affect the one infected pore. In fact, the entire area around the infection becomes red and inflamed. The body doesn't want to miss any of the infection, right? As other pores become red and irritated, they become enlarged and more vulnerable to additional bacterial attack. Inflammation of the skin can become a vicious cycle where the body's attempt to resolve infection makes it more vulnerable to more infection. This is why you will find acne on the list of inflammatory diseases.

The best way to prevent scarring from acne is to reduce inflammation at the acne site. It may sound convoluted, but there is the vicious cycle of acne—inflammation results from breakouts and also causes even more breakouts. If you want to limit acne and the scars associated with it, consider applying colostrum as a topical cream. Bovine colostrum is a powerful anti-inflammatory. In accompaniment with antioxidants and an anti-inflammatory diet, topical applications of colostrum on breakouts can speed healing, reduce local inflammation, and reduce the likelihood of acne scaring.

Previously we discussed the miraculous impact of colostrum on the immune system. There is research evidence to suggest that colostrum brings both overactive and underactive immune systems back into balance. Although research on colostrum and serious autoimmune disorders has yet to be conducted, topical applications of colostrum may offer new hope for some people with a skin condition called psoriasis. Psoriasis is an immune-modulated disease of the skin in which the immune system mistakenly attacks the skin. Although non-immune-modulated mechanisms for psoriasis have been proposed, the faulty immune explanation seems to be the most widely held. Psoriasis is a condition in which plaques of raised, thick skin appear at multiple sites of the body. In the case of psoriasis, the immune system attacks skin cells as if they were a pathological invader (like a virus) and emits faulty messenger chemicals telling skin cells to reproduce. This overproduction of skin cells results in patches of red or white hued skin called plaques. Killer T cells from your immune system swing into action, migrate to the skin, and stimulate the release of cytokines that cause inflammation. By returning the immune system to a happier homeostasis, attacks on the skin and symptoms of psoriasis could be reduced. Researchers at the Institute of Biotechnology in Australia suggest that the PRP found in colostrum has an inhibitory effect on autoimmune disorders such as multiple sclerosis [117]. If colostrum can have this PRP-mediated impact on multiple sclerosis, it could become a potent weapon against psoriasis that has an autoimmune dysfunction as its foundation.

Colostrum heals an inflamed bowel. Essentially, any part of the body that is consistently exposed to the outside world and its invaders (gut, lung, nose, and uterus) is designed to have cells that protect it. How do these protective mechanisms work? One example is that these parts of the body have cells that can produce lactoferrin in response to attack [113]. Researchers are beginning to suspect that lactoferrin could play a role in healing inflammatory gastrointestinal disorders like Crohn's disease and irritable bowel. First, we know that lactoferrin modulates gastric inflammation and that it is produced in the mucosa of the stomach lining [118,119]. We further know that lactoferrin interacts with receptors on gastric epithelial cells. Even further, we know that naturally occurring lactoferrin is elevated in the stool of people with inflammatory conditions of the bowel such as ulcerative colitis and Crohn's disease [111,120]. Even further still, mice studies have shown that administration of lactoferrin can reduce irritation of the gut after exposure to *Helicobacter felis* [121]. Put all of that evidence together, and we can conclude that the gut can absorb exogenous lactoferrin and thereby reduce the inflammation of its tissues.

In summary, the master anti-aging supplement has immense potential to be of benefit to people with treatment-resistant inflammatory bowel conditions. Clearly we need further human trials on lactoferrin and inflammatory disorders. Yet this supplement has the potential to offer healing to many people with these conditions. If you happen to have an inflammatory condition of the stomach or bowel, talk to your gastroenterologist to determine if you are a candidate for treatment with colostrum and lactoferrin.

In Conclusion

In my healing journey, I have refined my own diet to reduce inflammatory foods. When I gave up refined sugar, it felt like a food tragedy that I would never get over. If I hadn't been experiencing significant medical problems at the time, I would never have done it. I was a sugar addict and had to have something sweet with every meal — sweet cereal in the morning, cookies with lunch, and ice cream with dinner. I don't think that a day went by when I didn't have something with chocolate in it, and I poured sugar into all my beverages. My meals involved sugary rewards, and eating sweet things was one of the things that I used to make myself feel good. When I let go of refined sugar and restarted my diet to include only naturally occurring fruit sugars, everything tasted like cardboard. This went on for six weeks, and I didn't see how I was ever going to enjoy eating again. Then, suddenly, my withdrawal period was over. Fruit, which had always tasted lackluster, suddenly was bursting with newfound flavor. I could now taste the flavor behind the sweetness instead of only tasting that supersweet spike of cane sugar. This was only the beginning of my diet transformation, but it was my first step in taking care of me through good nutrition. Like any addict, I still get sugar cravings. But whereas I could only go a few hours without sugar in the past, now I limit myself to having something sweet every few months. Victory! When you are making major changes in your diet, keep in mind that the first six to eight weeks will be the hardest. After the withdrawal period, your experience of food will fundamentally change, and tastes will bloom in ways you cannot imagine now.

Another thing that I noticed when I incorporated more anti-inflammatory foods into my diet was that my food cravings declined. I felt less hungry, and my blood sugar levels seemed to be more stable. I attribute this to the fact that my food was more densely packed with nutrients. You feel hungry because your body is telling you that it doesn't have enough. But why is it that we can eat to the point of weight gain yet still get hunger messages telling us that we don't have enough? The answer lies in eating nutrient-dense foods. When your body tells you "I don't have enough" in the form of a hunger pang, it may not be talking about calories. In fact, it may be sending you hunger messages because it isn't getting enough nutrients. When we replace inflammatory, low-nutrient foods with anti-inflammatory, high-nutrient choices, we can feel less hungry — and when we feel less hungry, we are in a better position to prevent age-related weight gain.

CHAPTER 7

NEUTRACEUTICALS FOR TURNING BACK THE CLOCK

OUR NEXT AREA OF FOCUS is on nutritional support that you get from dietary supplements. Until the age of twenty-five, your body takes care of you; after twenty-five, you need to start taking care of your body. In the search for improved health and youthful stamina, most of us reach for vitamins, minerals, and antioxidants. The supplement industry is a multi-billion-dollar business. People, that's a lot of pills. You can't swing a virtual dead cat without hitting some Internet ad or pop-up about the latest, greatest thing in the supplement world. But which of these supplements actually work? How do we know that taking a supplement will lead to a reduction in the biological markers of aging?

This chapter reviews those supplements that have withstood long-term scientific scrutiny and those that have not. The health benefits of a small group of supplements are supported across time, researchers, and experimental conditions. You may be surprised at the list of the ones you should be taking. We also talk through some controversial issues surrounding supplements, including the free radical theory of aging and the harmful consequences of taking too many antioxidants. In this chapter, we discuss the evidence for essential fatty acids, the super juices, vitamin D, and antioxidants.

Laura Flynn Geissel, PhD

Essential Fatty Acids

I would like to discuss a class of neutraceuticals called essential fatty acids (EFAs). These are compounds that we need for good health; but because the body has no biochemical machinery for making its own, we have to ingest these fatty acids either from food or supplements. EFAs are modified by the body to make a number of compounds that affect inflammation, mood, and cellular signaling. How are EFAs anti-inflammatory? They are converted by the body into compounds called eicosanoids and endocannabinoids, which are cellular signaling compounds that tell the body to turn off the inflammatory alarm. For example, a daily diet of EFAs has been shown to reduce inflammatory allergic reactions in the nose [122]. Additionally, patients taking between one and eight grams of EFAs a day have shown improvement in various inflammatory disorders, including irritable bowel syndrome, rheumatoid arthritis, eczema, and psoriasis [123]. Just can't get away from our old friend inflammation, can we?

We have been studying the benefits of EFAs for decades. One specific organ in the body, the skin, has received a great deal of scientific study with respect to EFAs. Want to slow age-related changes in the skin? Consider adding EFAs to your diet. Because a large portion of skin aging can be attributed to the effects of sunlight (photoaging), there has been great scientific interest in how EFAs can reduce the effect of exposure to sunlight. The effects on skin exposed to UV radiation include epidermal thickening, DNA damage, and a reduction in collagen (the fluffy stuff that keeps skin bouncy and full-looking). When a particular essential fatty acid called eicosapentaenoic acid (EPA) was applied topically to the skin, the damage in response to UV radiation was reduced. Perhaps the most interesting finding in this study was that EPA-treated skin actually showed gains in two indicators that signify great skin: collagen and elastic fibers. Do you remember the growth factors we talked about in colostrum that are so good for skin repair? EPA actually improved these healthy skin markers by increasing levels of transforming growth factors [124]. Other studies on UV-induced skin damage have indicated that polyunsaturated fatty acids protect skin from changes due to UV radiation through its anti-inflammatory activity [125,126].

What about other types of skin problems such as wounds, eczema, and atopic dermatitis? EFAs can help all of these problems, too. When EFAs are applied to wounds, they stimulate early angiogenesis and promote wound repair. (Angiogenesis basically means that the EFAs help skin repair itself by increasing levels of skin growth factor.) EFAs act directly on certain genes to increase growth factors [127]. The authors of this study even recommend EFAs as an alternative to gene therapy and topical hormones for complex wounds. Another study on atopic dermatitis showed that EFAs are as good or better than topical steroids for healing skin lesions. Although effective, repeated applications of topical steroids can lead to skin thinning and skin breakage. Steroids are one of those mixed-bag treatments for the skin. If topical EFAs can do the work of steroids, dermatologists do not have to worry about these alarming side effects [128].

The name *essential fatty acid* really captures the importance of these compounds for the body; they are essential. The brain can't even develop in the fetal and postnatal periods without them [129]. EFAs even help the brain in old age. Older people who supplement their diet with EFAs have a decreased risk of dementia and Alzheimer's disease [130]. As a former counseling psychologist, I really can't leave the topic of EFAs without briefly commenting on the topic of mood disorders. EFAs boost mood, just like they boost cognition. Women are up to 50 percent more likely than men to experience a depressive episode in their lifetimes. Some authors explain this difference by citing differences in hormones and organic brain chemistry, whereas others focus on the perceived marginalization of women in our society. As a former counseling psychologist, I am also acutely aware of the psychic pain that depression exerts on many people. Although antidepressant medications work wonders for some people, they just are not right for others. Either these medications do not restore the delicate balance of neurotransmitters in the brain or the side effects make them intolerable. If you have tried antidepressants but the side effects are just too much for you, you are not alone—and it's not because you are a weak person. These medications are very powerful, with equally powerful side effects. If you talk to any honest psychiatrist, he will tell you that we have only the most general idea of how these medications work.

With all of that said, the field of psychiatry is currently exploring how EFAs can work as well or better than antidepressants without the risk of side effects. Researchers conducting a recent meta-analysis (a study in which published data sets are analyzed rather than developing an original data set) of studies evaluating the role of omega-3 fatty acids concluded that there are sufficient data favoring omega-3 supplementation for patients with a depressive mood disorder [131]. They concluded that EFAs have few side effects and are neuroprotective. Another study on treatment-resistant depression concluded that omega-3 fatty acid supplementation results in a marked improvement in mood symptoms for depressed or bipolar patients [132]. The researchers observed that clinical improvement is proportional to improvement achieved via medication with either lithium or lamotrigine. Finally, supplementation of omega-3 fatty acids may also be helpful for anxiety disorders. Two recent studies have documented the prevention of posttraumatic stress disorder symptoms by administering EFAs after a traumatic event [133,134].

So, if EFAs are that good for us, how do we get them? One of the best ways to obtain EFAs is through a supplement of fish oil. Unfortunately, it's almost impossible to eat enough fish-based meals to get the EFAs you need. But how much fish oil should you take? First, make sure that you choose a supplement company that conducts rigorous testing for heavy metals. If you take a supplement with high mercury content, you could be hurting yourself as much as you are helping yourself with your fish oil supplement. The fatty acids in fish oil are abbreviated as EPA and DHA. Experts debate how much fish oil you need to take. In general, look for a ratio of DHA to EPA that is 2:1. The recommended amount of fish oil that experts discuss is one to three grams per day. Studies showing the efficacy of fish oil on participants range up to five grams a day. For general use, stick to one to three grams a day with doses on the higher end if your desired outcome is improved mental health symptoms. Taking more than this should be conducted under the advice of your medical professional. Remember, fish oil is a blood thinner — this is partially why it is good for the cardiovascular system. Therefore you should ask your doctor if you have any health conditions for which a blood-thinning effect could cause complications. For example, you cannot take fish oil for at least two weeks prior to surgery because it interferes with blood clotting.

THE SUPER JUICES

In recent years, the scientific community has been building up a wealth of data supporting the use of medicinal berries and fruits to improve well-being and halt intrinsic age-related changes. The four fruits discussed in this section include pomegranate, goji, mangosteen, and açai. Incorporating one of these fruits, typically as a whole fruit juice, into your diet can have a profound effect on your energy, well-being, and overall health. Most of the juices discussed here have overlapping effects on human health. This is because the active ingredients in pomegranate, mangosteen, goji, and açai are similar. However, there are some slight differences. As you browse this section, choose the super juice that sounds the best for your situation and add one to your diet after clearing it with your general practitioner. The scientific data provided in each section have been summarized in the following table. Take a look at the table and talk to your doctor about which of these you can take. Bear in mind that many of these juices interfere with certain medications, such as warfarin.

The Super Juice Comparison Chart

Healing effect	Açai	Mangosteen	Pomegranate	Goji
Supports innate antioxidant system	Yes	Yes	Yes	Yes
Anti-inflammatory	Yes	Yes	Yes	Yes
Weight management	Yes	Yes	Yes	No evidence found
Cardiovascular health	Yes	No evidence found	Yes	Yes
Anticancer	Yes	Yes	Yes	Yes
General immunity	Yes	Yes	Yes	Yes
Anti-aging	Yes	Yes	Yes	Yes

Açai. The açai is a type of palm tree, also called *Euterpe oleracea*. It was originally cultivated for hearts of palm, a white, fibrous center that is considered by many to be a gourmet vegetable. Today açai is mainly grown in Central and South America for its fruit, known as the açai berry. The berry is a small, dark purple fruit that looks similar to the grape. The main source of the many health benefits of açai are the polyphenols contained in the skin and the flesh of the fruit. The fruit also contains low levels of another well-known antioxidant, resveratrol (discussed in a later section). Let's take a look at some of the evidence supporting the "super juice" status of açai.

Toxicology studies on mice have shown that açai has no toxic effects. In fact, it has a healing and protective effect when cells are exposed to chemicals that cause DNA damage. In this study, mice who were administered three grams of açai per kilogram of body weight were significantly protected against DNA damage in the liver and kidneys [135]. The authors concluded that these beneficial effects are due to the phytochemicals in the fruit. So are you thinking about supplementing with açai juice? Unfortunately, these positive attributes do not extend to the taste of açai. As the percentage of açai goes up in a sample of juice, the perceived favorableness of the taste goes down. In addition, as people become more dissatisfied with the taste, their ratings of the perceived health benefits of açai also go down [136]. But just because it tastes bad doesn't mean it isn't good for you.

Most of the literature that you will read on açai talks about its antioxidant benefits. However, these well-positioned marketing strategies fail to mention that the compounds from açai do not enter cells, where much of the free radicals in the body are produced. On the bright side, I did discover research documenting that açai can offer support to the body's innate antioxidant system. When administered in an animal model, açai increased the activity of glutathione in neutralizing free radicals [137]. Not bad, açai.

Açai is also a potent anti-inflammatory agent. Administration of açai can reduce the body's tendency to produce cytokines, messenger proteins that the body uses to trigger an inflammatory reaction. Concentrations of cytokines in the body can increase by a thousand times in response to injury or infection. In fact, açai can reduce multiple biomarkers of inflammation [138]. One example of a chronic inflammatory symptom is chronic pain. In a clinical study, patients with chronic pain and limited range of motion were given 120 milliliters of mixed açai fruit juice for twelve weeks. At the end of the study, participants in the juice group reported a reduction in pain, an increase in range of motion, and an increased ability to engage in daily life activities [139]. Other studies using animal models have suggested that açai can even reduce inflammation in the brain [140] and inflammatory biomarkers in the lungs in response to cigarette smoke [141]. All of this research points to the fact that açai can help with intrinsic aging as well as attacks on the body from the environment.

Much of the promotion of açai also has to do with using this supplement for weight loss. Actually, there is actual scientific data to back up the use of açai as part of a sensible weight management program. In one study, ten obese adults were given one hundred grams of açai pulp twice daily for a period of one month. These people exhibited a reduction in cholesterol and in two markers of weight problems, including fasting glucose and insulin [142]. Another study using an animal model indicated that organisms given açai were more likely to survive on a fatally high-fat diet [143].

Other work on açai has supported claims that this supplement helps to improve cardiovascular health and acts as an anticancer agent. With regard to cardiovascular health, açai acts on the signaling system that tells the body to reduce its production of cholesterol [144]. It also induces an antihypertensive effect while preventing changes in blood vessel tissues associated with hypertension [145]. Other work has supported previous findings that açai improves lipid profiles and reduces atherosclerosis [146]. Finally, açai has been shown to reduce clinical markers of leukemia [147], bladder cancer [148], and colon cancer [149].

Mangosteen. The mangosteen is a medicinal fruit that originated in Indonesia. The purple fruit comes from a tree and is cultivated in Southeast Asia and South America. Most people think of the mango when they first begin to learn about the purple mangosteen. However, the two bear little similarity, except in name. The tree on which the fruit grows is a type of tropical evergreen, while the fruit consists of a hard purple rind surrounding a white, fleshy interior. Mangosteen is available for purchase as a juice and provides the user with a host of systemic health benefits. When choosing a mangosteen product, look for a juice that has been processed using the whole fruit. Most of the health benefits from the fruit come from the xanthonoids, such as mangostin, that are in the dark purple rind. Your mangosteen juice should be processed using extracts from the rind to have the most health benefits. For the rest of this section, we will talk about these benefits, which range from controlling weight gain to stopping cancers.

The major active ingredients of the mangosteen are two xanthones called α-mangostin and γ-mangostin. But if we know what the bioactive components are, why not just take supplements made from these extracts? This question gets to the argument for whole food-sourced nutrients over supplements and synthetically sourced compounds. (We will discuss this more in the antioxidant section of the chapter.) We know that it is a general rule that whole food sources of nutrients are more readily available to the body as compared to supplement sources. With this in mind, researchers validated the fact that the xanthones from the mangosteen fruit juice were converted more readily into bioavailable, usable compounds than xanthones extracted from the fruit. Thus oral administration of the juice provided higher levels of the active forms of the xanthones than direct injection of these compounds [150].

Mangosteen helps the body improve along a number of specific health indicators. First, supplementation with mangosteen juice can help with age-related weight gain. In one study, sixty overweight subjects were divided into either a mangosteen treatment group or placebo. Subjects were given an identical diet and began a mild exercise program of walking five days a week. After an eight-week period, the body mass index and waist circumference were significantly lower in the treatment group as compared to placebo. The researchers were able to associate weight loss in the treatment group to a number of biomarkers specifically related to changes in weight. For example, administration of mangosteen increased expression of adiponectin [151]. Adiponectin is a protein-based hormone; when it is high, the percentage of body fat goes down.

Second, supplementation with mangosteen can also help the body fight off invasive bacteria. Antibiotic-resistant bacteria are considered to be one of the four horsemen of the apocalypse for the modern medical community. As our antibiotics begin to fail more rapidly, we need to introduce other supporting therapies that can prevent or help stop an infection. Mangosteen has the potential to be one of these therapies. Researchers used an antibiotic-resistant strain of staphylococcus isolated from the eye and exposed it to xanthones from mangosteen. Although

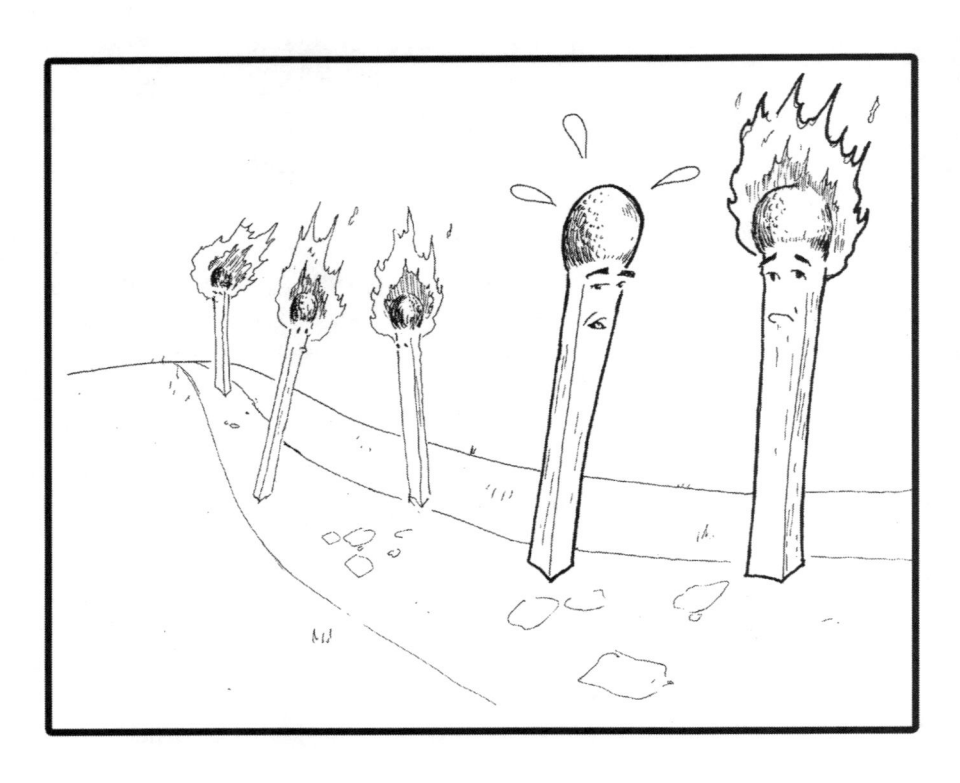

"What's wrong with you, Francis?"
"I'm on an anti-inflammatory diet."

this bug was resistant to the antibiotic methicillin, it exhibited no resistance to α-mangostin and was killed in a number of minutes. Electron microscopy showed that cell death was due to α-mangostin's ability to break the cell membrane [152]. Other studies have demonstrated the activity of xanthones from mangosteen to kill multi-drug-resistant bacteria [153].

Mangosteen is also a potent anti-inflammatory. In a previous chapter, we discussed the nature of inflammation and why it is bad for the body. Remember, acute inflammation is designed to rid the body of an allergen or pathogen. Chronic inflammation sets in when these efforts have failed. It is highly likely that nutraceuticals with anti-inflammatory properties help the body to more easily rid itself of invaders, or these compounds may impact the cellular signaling pathways to reduce the body's reactivity to harmless stimuli such as dust and pollen. Studies have shown that the main xanthones from mangosteen, α-mangostin and γ-mangostin, reduce the pathophysiological markers of allergic asthma. These asthma-related changes in response to mangosteen included reduced movement of inflammatory cells into the airways and reduced airway hyperresponsiveness. The authors concluded that mangosteen may have potential as a supporting therapy for asthma [154]. A number of other studies have been conducted showing the anti-inflammatory activity of mangosteen [155,156,157,158]. When your cells go through an inflammatory cycle, they actually show increased ability to make use of the xanthones from mangosteen [159].

How do the active ingredients in mangosteen exert their activity to assist the body? The scientific community is still debating the mechanism of action for xanthones in mangosteen. However, one study suggests that mangosteen may support the body's own natural antioxidant system, which is based on glutathione inside cells. In this study, cells were exposed to various doses of α-mangostin and were then challenged by a toxic free radical generator called ferrous sulfate. As levels of α-mangostin went up, the levels of reduced glutathione (glutathione that has already given away its electron to a free radical) went down. This means that the body was able to use mangosteen to reduce free radicals outside of cells, thus preserving glutathione inside cells, which reduces free radicals that are made by the cellular machinery [160].

Finally, mangosteen has shown great potential in numerous studies as an anticancer therapy. Mangosteen has been shown to induce cancer cell death and to retard the spread of cancer cells in studies conducted in the lab and in living organisms [161]. Mangosteen is so effective because it can target many, not just one, signaling pathway, telling cancer cells to destruct. These signaling pathways are special chemical messengers that tell cells to divide, grow, and die. Mangosteen has been shown to reduce colon cancer tumor size [162] and to prevent colon cancer cell invasion and migration [163]. Remember, cancerous changes happen in the body all the time, and these events increase with age. By adding a xanthone-based therapy, your immune system gets a much-needed foot soldier for the battle. Finally, mangosteen has also been shown to inhibit all stages of the cancer cell life cycle for human skin cancer [164] and bladder cancer [165].

Pomegranate. The pomegranate has been cultivated and harvested as a nutritional food since ancient times. The fruit consists of groupings of juice-filled sacs in a hard husk. Today, it is grown throughout the East, including in the Mediterranean, the Middle East, India, and Africa. Research on this super juice has suggested positive benefits for heart health, diabetes, and certain forms of cancer [166]. Toxicology studies have shown that pomegranate juice and extracts are proven to be safe [167]. Most of the promotion by the alternative health and supplement community has to do with the presence of polyphenols in the fruit. It has been believed that these compounds boost health through their antioxidant properties.

However, the pomegranate may be more mysterious than previously thought. Using a biomarker of the moment-by-moment antioxidant capacity of the blood called nonenzymatic antioxidant capacity, researchers at the Antioxidant Research Laboratory in Rome, Italy, have presented some confusing facts about pomegranate. Polyphenols are believed to be the antioxidant powerhouse of pomegranate. Yet these researchers found that higher concentrations of polyphenols in the body are not correlated with an increase in the antioxidant capacity of the blood. These authors also described a low rate of absorption for polyphenols and raised general concerns about the degree to which pomegranate contributes to health through the mechanism of reducing free radicals [168]. Despite the hype, free radical reduction may not be the main pathway through which pomegranate contributes to health.

Even though we may not know how it happens, the pomegranate has been shown to have positive broad-spectrum effects on human health. In one study, patients were given one hundred cubic centimeters of pomegranate juice three times weekly for a year. The researchers evaluated participants on inflammatory markers, rates of hospitalization due to infection, and progression of plaque in the arteries. First, the pomegranate juice group exhibited a reduction in inflammatory markers as compared to placebo controls. Second, the pomegranate juice group had a significantly lower incidence of infection that resulted in hospitalization. Finally, 25 percent of the pomegranate group showed an improvement in artery health, while 50 percent of the placebo group showed progression of arterial plaque [169]. Thus a moderate amount of pomegranate improved cardiovascular health, general immunity, and inflammation.

Many other studies have also demonstrated the anti-inflammatory properties of pomegranate. In the gut, polyphenols are neutralized into compounds called urolithins. It is believed that it is these compounds that then go to work to reduce systemic and gut-related inflammation [170,171]. For example, ten milliliters per day of pomegranate reduced biochemical markers of arthritic inflammation for patients with rheumatoid arthritis [172]. Pomegranate may be an excellent complementary therapy to reduce inflammation throughout the body.

Pomegranate has also been marketed as a weight loss tool

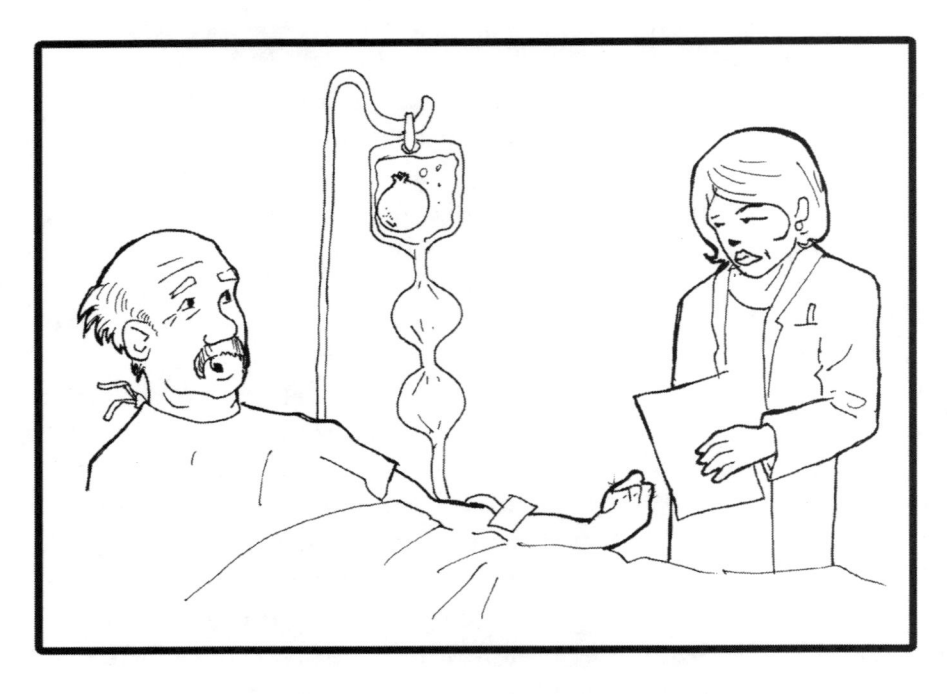

"Hey, Doc, I'm all for whole food sources, but how are these pomegranates going to get through this needle?"

to reduce age-related weight gain. Interestingly, this assertion has been borne out by the scientific literature. Supplementation with the pomegranate has shown to enhance fat reduction [173]. Although pomegranate did not modify how much insulin was secreted by the body, it did help people in the pomegranate treatment group to avoid increases in weight, body mass index, and fat mass as compared to a placebo group [174]. Thus pomegranate can help prevent a natural inclination for age-related adiposy. However, if you decide to supplement with pomegranate for weight loss, be sure that you watch your caloric intake. Juice from the pomegranate can significantly add to the amount of calories that you consume each day and interfere with your weight loss goals.

Finally, pomegranate has shown some promise as an anticancer agent. Two studies have been conducted specifically with breast cancer. In each, pomegranate was shown to interfere with some attribute of the breast cancer cell life cycle. In one study, pomegranate was shown to interfere with the protein-copying mechanism in breast cancer cells, reducing their ability to proliferate [175]. In another study, pomegranate was shown to affect estrogen receptors, depleting breast cancer cells of needed estrogen [176]. What about men? Pomegranate has also been shown to reduce proliferation of prostate cancer cells and pancreatic cancer cells [177,178].

Before beginning significant supplementation with pomegranate, talk to your doctor. Pomegranate can interfere with the activity of certain medications such as warfarin [179].

Goji. The final super juice that we discuss in this chapter is called goji berry. Also called wolfberry, this berry is the fruit of the *Lycium barbarum* plant. This plant was originally cultivated in southeastern Europe and Asia. Today, the majority of the commercially available fruit comes from China. Goji berry is considered a super fruit because of its broad benefits and because only small amounts are necessary to get these benefits. Goji is considered a broad-spectrum anti-aging supplement, and its benefits hit multiple systems in the body. Goji has also been shown to be a pharmacological agent in halting the progression of age-related diseases, including diabetes and atherosclerosis [180].

Supplementation with goji berry can improve your general well-being. While most of the research on goji comes out of China, where the fruit is grown, one study conducted in the West has demonstrated the broad benefits of this berry when consumed as a juice. Healthy adults were given either a placebo control drink or 120 milliliters of goji juice for fourteen days. Participants in the goji group reported an amazing diversity in improvements as compared to controls. These improvements included access to energy, athletic skills, quality of sleep, concentration, ability to relax, and perceptions of health, contentment, and happiness. Those taking goji reduced their fatigue, stress, and gastrointestinal dysfunction [181].

Throughout this book, we have been talking about the importance of reducing inflammation to enhance biochemical performance of the body. Like the other super juices, goji is a powerful anti-inflammatory. When it is infected with a virus, for example, the body activates its inflammatory processes to clear the infection. One study conducted with mice showed that goji reduced the symptoms and intensity of influenza infection. Infected mice given goji did not exhibit as much infection-related weight loss and lung dysfunction. How does goji juice accomplish such feats? Goji decreases the levels of chemical messengers that the body uses to trigger inflammation and increases the effectiveness of killer T cells, so it both boosts immune activity and reduces chemical messengers that cause inflammation [182].

Many other studies have investigated processes by which goji can reduce inflammation and speed healing of the body. In one study, rats were given goji and a chemical that caused liver damage. Goji berry protected the rats against cell death and reduced inflammatory messenger chemicals in the liver. Because their livers were protected from cell death and inflammation, those in the treatment group did not show as much fibrosis of the liver [183]. Aside from protecting the liver, goji can also protect neurons in the nervous system from chemical damage [184] and skin cells from UV damage [185].

Anything that is good for your immune system has anti-aging properties. The immune system conducts all of the repair processes that keep the body in a youthful, healthy state. As we age, our natural antioxidant capacity declines. Goji berry supports our own antioxidant enzymes and stops age-related decline of the immune system. In one study, goji was shown to restore the power of the immune system in aging mice [186]. In this study, an influenza vaccine was given to 150 elderly Chinese subjects, while half of the participants were given 13.7 grams of goji per day. Older persons given goji showed higher levels of antibodies that were specific to influenza. In other words, people in the goji group responded more strongly to the vaccine and acquired greater protection from future influenza infection [187]. These findings were replicated in aging mice; those mice given goji showed a significant increase in immune system markers that tend to decrease with age [188]. Another study using older adults given fresh goji berries indicated that participants increased the number of lymphocytes, interleukin-2, and immunoglobulin G as compared to older adults not eating goji for thirty days [189]. We can conclude that goji increases major indicators of the immune system including (1) number of white blood cells, (2) immune signaling proteins that direct white blood cells, and (3) basic building blocks for antibodies.

Goji berry has also shown promise as an anticancer agent. In one study, administration of goji berry was shown to increase immune signaling in the fight against one type of cancer [190]. If we can increase the body's ability to talk to its immune system about the presence of cancer cells, then we stand a better change to eradicate those cells. Another study on prostate cancer showed that goji increased programmed cell death of cancer cells, while reducing tumor growth and weight [191].

Finally, when you consider adding goji to your diet, talk to your doctor about whether it is right for you. Goji can interfere with the activity of certain medications such as warfarin [192].

Vitamin D

When we think about "getting our vitamins," we generally think about the big three: vitamin C, vitamin E, and the B vitamins. But there is another letter in the mix that you might want to think about first. Addressing a vitamin D deficiency is one of the best things you can do for your health as you age. My holistic physician told me that a vitamin D deficiency is as bad for you as smoking two packs of cigarettes a day. Your body can make some vitamin D when exposed to sunlight; however, there are two problems with this approach. Most of us working in office environments do not get enough sun exposure to make enough vitamin D. Even if you have a lifestyle in which you are exposed to the sun, UV exposure can cause photoaging and skin cancer. It is recommended to close the gap on vitamin D insufficiency with an oral supplement to circumvent these problems.

Multiple studies have shown that people with a vitamin D deficiency are more likely to die early from a variety of causes as compared to their nondeficient peers. One study on approximately ten thousand older German adults indicated that vitamin D deficiency was linked to death from cardiovascular problems, cancer, and diseases of the respiratory tract [193]. Unfortunately, a number of people have a hidden vitamin D deficiency. One meta-analysis looked at data from studies conducted in Latin America and found that 24 percent of preschoolers and 10 percent of adults were deficient [194]. Another study conducted in Canada found insufficiency in vitamin D among 26 percent of adults. Risks may be even higher for people with darker skin and for pregnant women [195].

When vitamin D runs low, we can run into a variety of health problems. This vitamin supports the immune system and tells it what to do. For example, among people with allergic diseases (where the immune system attacks things that it should ignore), vitamin D deficiency was associated with higher levels of allergic response [196]. In this book, we have talked over and over about the dangers of inflammation. People with low vitamin D also have increased levels of inflammation [197]. Proper amounts of vitamin D reduce unnecessary and unwanted inflammation, allowing the immune system to focus its work where it is needed [198]. Low vitamin D has been linked to illness in chronically ill children and adults as well as to cardiovascular problems, problems with metabolism, and impaired lung function [199].

Fortunately, when you supplement with vitamin D, immune system dysfunction goes away, risk of infection drops, and risk of death declines significantly [200]. Vitamin D also supports the body when it is dealing with the "Big C," or cancer. In one study, researchers assessed vitamin D for patients with malignant melanoma; low levels of vitamin D in the blood were associated with poorer outcome and thicker melanomas [201]. This magical hormone has been shown to induce the death of cancer cells and inhibit their growth. The authors of this work concluded that vitamin D is a safe, low-cost, and effective method for breast cancer prevention [202].

In conclusion, talk to your doctor. Although your skin can make vitamin D when exposed to sunlight, chances are that you are not getting enough. Your doctor can check your levels with a simple blood test and recommend a supplement dose for you.

The Good and the Bad about Antioxidants

The antioxidant supplement craze can be traced back to the research and theory of one man: Denham Harmon. In 1956, he proposed the basis of what would later be known as the free radical theory of aging. A free radical is an unstable molecule. Basically, it needs to grab an electron from another molecule, turning this second molecule into a free radical, and the damage continues in a chain reaction. This process is also referred to as oxidative stress, or the giving and taking of electrons. Think of the wall of your cells like the walls of a brick building. A free radical comes along and steals a brick from the wall of your house. To fill the hole, another brick is stolen from somewhere else. Over time, this continual shuffling of bricks weakens or breaks the wall. Antioxidants stop this chain reaction by their ability to donate an electron, while remaining stable themselves.

To understand how antioxidants really work, we need first to understand cellular oxidation. When you examine the atoms that make up your cells, you will find pairs of electrons that travel around the center of the atom. Electrons, like people, prefer to be in pairs. In the process of oxidation, an atom becomes unstable when it loses one or more of its paired electrons. This atom is now unhappy. So it goes out and tries to steal an electron from another atom or dump its extra electron in another atom, causing this new atom to become unstable. This new, unhappy atom wants to do something with its unpaired electron, and so a domino effect of electron transfer occurs. These unhappy atoms are called free radicals, and many experts believe that the domino effect of electron depositing and stealing is the source of all cellular aging.

Antioxidants are what come in to stop the domino effect and neutralize free radicals. They basically work by giving electrons to the free radical and returning it to a happy, stable state. For example, vitamin C uses other electrons in its molecule to take turns filling in for the electron it donated so that it does not need to steal from a different molecule. What if we didn't have free radicals to stop this process? We see oxidation outside the body all the time. The example of a rusting car gives you a very clear picture of what oxidation from free radicals might look like on the cellular level. Rust is a process in which an electron from iron is transferred to an oxygen molecule. Without antioxidants to shut down this process, it's a quick trip to a body that is rusted from the inside out. Harmon came to believe that antioxidants could extend life through biochemical means and that the source of all aging is damage from free radicals.

Many studies have linked free radical damage with either aging or disease. For example, one study showed that the formation of free radicals increases in rats as they get older [203]. One particular variety of mouse, the Ames Dwarf mouse, lives longer and has better oxidative stress resistance than other types of mice. This long-lived mouse genetically produces lower amounts of reactive oxygen species than other mice, suggesting that a lower amount of free radicals may be the cause of its long life [204]. These findings also seem to extend to humans in studies of endothelial dysfunction in blood vessels that showed correlation with vessel inflammation and oxidative stress [205].

But what is the mechanism by which free radicals cause damage that we would define as aging? One possible mechanism is that the electron stealing by free radicals can cause the base-pair molecules in your DNA to fuse. When this DNA strand is copied to make a new cell, this error in the gene can be passed along to all new cells until enough damaged cells exist to cause a problem. If the fused gene codes for an important enzyme or chemical messenger, this type of free radical damage can be catastrophic. For example, this fusing of DNA molecules can lead to cancerous growths [206]. Another type of fusing can occur between fat and protein molecules. When this happens on the surface of the skin, one area of the skin gets chemically bonded to another area. These "stuck" areas appear visually as wrinkles. One of the reasons that dermatologists recommend topical antioxidants is that they can prevent this type of free radical that leads to wrinkles on the surface of the skin [207].

Although Harmon showed that antioxidants could extend the relative life-span of some organisms, such as rats, mice, and fruit flies, he was unable to demonstrate that antioxidants could extend maximum life-span. That means that if the maximum life-span of a mouse is three years, then antioxidants can make that mouse more likely to live for three years, but not for longer. Harmon felt that he had to modify his theory. He then proposed the mitochondrial theory of aging. To understand the function of mitochondria, let's talk briefly about fractals. The theory of fractal structure tells us that the structural pattern that can be observed at the macro level must also be present at the micro

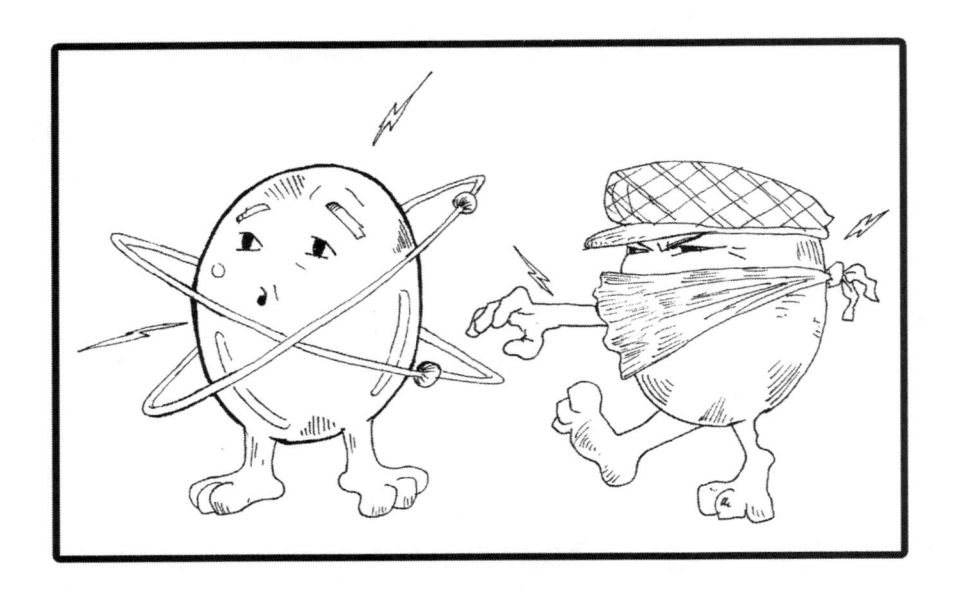

Free radicals . . . the white collar criminals of the body.

level. Therefore the large organ structures that we observe in the body must also be observable in the smallest unit of the body: the cell. To understand what the mitochondria do, think of these bean-shaped bags of stuff like the stomach of the cell. In the stomach, food is broken down into glucose (a sugar) that can be used for energy. This glucose is then transported inside the cell, where it is converted into a molecule called ATP by the mitochondria. ATP is then distributed throughout the cell as a molecule that holds the energy of glucose for biochemical processes. The little organelles called the mitochondria is essentially the power plant of the cell. But like your stomach produces waste that you later excrete, the mitochondria also produce waste. In the process of making ATP, a variety of free radical species are formed inside cells as a waste product of the chemical reaction. So, Harmon revised his theory to say that mitochondria are damaged by free radicals and also produce them. It is this endogenous production of free radicals that is the source of aging. Unfortunately, antioxidants that we take orally cannot enter the mitochondria. Harmon concluded that it is the amount of damage to the mitochondria that determines life-span [208].

Left unchecked, oxidation from free radical damage can eventually cause cell death, and that is why the body has so many redundant mechanisms for stopping it. Unfortunately, life on Earth requires oxygen for basic chemical processes, but oxygen has a high potential to turn into free radicals. In fact, it can morph into one of three different types of free radicals, superoxide anion, hydrogen peroxide, or hydroxyl radical. These unhappy oxygen molecules then do damage to other molecules as they try to borrow electrons that they are missing. Antioxidants help us by preventing these reactive oxygen species from forming or by neutralizing them before they can do much damage [209]. Some of the most important antioxidants to the human body include uric acid [210], vitamin C [211], glutathione [212], vitamin E [213], and melatonin [214]. Let's talk about a few antioxidants in more detail and examine whether the free radical theory of aging has held up over time.

Resveratrol. If you are up on your antioxidant literature, chances are that you have heard of resveratrol. The proposed health benefits of resveratrol are numerous and include cancer prevention, cardioprotection, diabetes prevention, anti-inflammatory effects, and antiviral effects. Numerous food sources of resveratrol exist, including red wine and Japanese knotweed. In one controversial finding, resveratrol was even shown to extend the life-span of worms [215]. Is there anything this natural phenol can't do? Resveratrol may also be the reason for the *French paradox,* the epidemiological finding that the French diet of heavy cream sauces and saturated fat does not seem to increase heart disease for the French [216]. However, when we look closely at the research on resveratrol, we find that the efficacy of this supplement may not be as cut and dry as we thought. First, people are not worms, and so we don't know if the life-extending impact on worms will transfer to humans. I don't know about you, but I like to think of myself as being very different from a worm. That said, there are quite a few studies showing that resveratrol works against cancer in various animals [217]. However, at the time of this publication, there have been no studies showing that resveratrol alone inhibits cancer activity in humans. I was able to find a few studies showing that resveratrol can potentiate the anticancer activity of other treatments, such as quercetin [218], and other similar polyphenols [219] and that it enhances the effect of radiation [220]. But how large is the effect size for resveratrol alone? That, we just don't know yet.

I want to share a few more issues with resveratrol that I think are relevant to anyone who is considering taking it. For the moment, we don't know how resveratrol affects the body in the long term. One author has theorized that because the chemical structure of resveratrol is similar to a phytoestrogen, this compound could stimulate the proliferation of breast cancer cells [221]. If you are a woman with a history of breast cancer in your family, I really don't recommend this supplement for you.

What seems to be lacking most in research with resveratrol and humans is a good delivery method. When you take a pill of resveratrol, approximately 70 percent is absorbed by the stomach. However, only 1 percent of what is absorbed is available for your body to use because of the activity of the liver and other biochemical processes, which break it down [222]. After taking a pill of the stuff, only trace amounts can be found in the blood. When absorbed through the stomach, the liver breaks it down before it can be used. The strongest anticancer activity for resveratrol has been found for tumors that it can touch, such as tumors in the digestive tract or skin [223]. When taking resveratrol, you have to consider whether it can get to the part of the body you want to affect. You also need to consider whether you can actually absorb enough resveratrol to reach the same serum doses that were used to demonstrate efficacy in animal model studies. In sum, it's unlikely that taking pills of resveratrol can get enough of the stuff into the body to prevent cancer in organs beyond the skin and digestive tract [224].

The best way to absorb resveratrol is through the cheeks and gums. If you are up on your Internet ads, you have probably heard that drinking red wine responsibly has been associated with a reduced risk of heart disease [225]. Many studies have suggested a fact about resveratrol: it is the active ingredient about red wine that provides its cardioprotective effect [226]. Research on the specific resveratrol found in red wine has demonstrated multiple pathways to this effect, including reducing the aggregation of platelets [227] and inhibiting the spread of vascular smooth muscle [228]. Although these later studies are by reputable authors, the author who first proposed the link between resveratrol and cardioprotection was found guilty of research fraud in 2012. This means that he falsified his findings and the work had to be retracted. Regardless, taking resveratrol in pill form is unlikely to provide the healing effect for which you are looking. Look for a liquid product that you can hold in your mouth or a resveratrol gum. Perhaps all the wine aficionados have it right: sip, swish, and spit.

Glutathione. Did you know that your body makes its own antioxidants? One of the most important antioxidants that your body uses to reduce or neutralize free radicals is one that you make inside your own cells. It's called glutathione. Glutathione has been all over the news lately, and many top athletes get weekly injections of glutathione to reach peak physical performance. If you go out to the supplement market, you will find many glutathione products ranging from tablets to nasal sprays. Unfortunately, your body does not absorb glutathione very well from these delivery methods. It is a highly unstable compound, meaning that it can easily break down to a nonactive from between the time that it is produced and the time that you take it. Glutathione is a powerful antioxidant, and it is looking for any excuse to give away one of its electrons. By the time it gets to you from an over-the-counter source, much of its neutralizing power has already been used up. The most reliable ways to increase your levels of glutathione are either to increase the amount of glutathione building blocks you ingest or get injections of it from your holistic physician. By taking a product called NAC (N-acetyl cysteine), you can increase the bioavailability of the building blocks your cells use to make their own glutathione. Bovine colostrum, the master anti-aging supplement, also supplies the body with the basic building blocks for glutathione. Talk to your doctor about whether supplementation with NAC or glutathione injections are right for you.

Why is glutathione important? For one thing, low glutathione levels have been linked to chronic illness. In one study that compared chronically ill patients to healthy controls, glutathione levels were about 60 percent lower in the ill group. These low levels were true for total glutathione as well as the amount of glutathione that had already given away electrons to free radicals [229]. Another study looked at the converse: whether healthy people are more likely to have higher levels of glutathione. Using a community-based sample of the elderly, these researchers showed that higher glutathione levels were associated with a lower number of illnesses. In fact, higher glutathione was linked to a number of pro-health indicators, including higher self-ratings of overall health, lower cholesterol, lower body mass, and lower blood pressure [230]. Help for critically ill patients could come in the form of supplementation with NAC. Critically ill patients given nutrition loaded with cysteine do show improved ability to make their own glutathione [231]. We do not understand the exact mechanism of activity yet, but it seems that it is easier to get seriously ill when glutathione levels are low. We will talk later about the fact that most orally administered antioxidants cannot enter your cells and are therefore not able to reduce free radicals inside cells. Perhaps the protective mechanism of this antioxidant has to do with its ability to reduce free radicals inside cells when your body makes its own.

Finally, glutathione is good brain food. The scientific literature charts a clear path indicating that those with Parkinson's disease have a glutathione deficiency in the brain. Conversely, when Parkinson's patients were given intravenous glutathione, all participants improved with a clinically significant decline in markers of disability [232]. Levels of glutathione in the brain have also been shown to be lower for people diagnosed with schizophrenia. When participants were given a dietary supplement of the basic building blocks for glutathione (NAC), their schizophrenic symptoms improved. The study's authors concluded that NAC may be an effective supporting treatment for schizophrenia [233].

Vitamin C, vitamin E, beta-carotene, and vitamin A. The clinical picture for the efficacy of common antioxidants is more complicated than most people know. The father of the free radical theory of aging posited that there are limits to the amount of anti-aging protection that we can get from antioxidants [208]. Because we cannot get antioxidants into the mitochondria, there is a limit to how much we can do to prevent aging from free radicals that originate inside the cells. Although many studies have shown the health benefits of antioxidants, just as many studies have shown no benefit or actual harm. For example, when you stop the roundworm (*Caenorhabditis elegans*) from making its own endogenous antioxidant (superoxide dismutase), you *increase* its life-span [234]. In other words, these worms live longer when they have less circulating antioxidants. Other researchers have replicated these findings with the roundworm and have called into question the widespread use of antioxidants in humans [235]. But what about humans? Take a look at the following list of studies showing no positive benefit for antioxidants:

- *Antioxidants increased cancer rates.* In this study, smokers, former smokers, and workers exposed to asbestos were given beta-carotene and vitamin A daily for four years. Antioxidant use did not reduce their rates of cancer as compared to placebo controls. After examining 388 new cases of lung cancer for those enrolled in the study, the antioxidant group actually had a relatively higher cancer risk [236].

- *Antioxidants did not prevent cancer.* A study looked at lung cancer rates for male smokers on a five- to eight-year supplementation period. There was no reduction in lung cancer rates for this population of 29,133 smokers who took fifty IU per day of vitamin E or twenty milligrams per day of beta-carotene. In fact, a higher rate of lung cancer was reported for men who took beta-carotene alone [237].

- *Antioxidants increased death rates.* This study looked at how vitamin E performed across nineteen different clinical trials for 135,967 participants. Eleven of those nineteen clinical studies used high-dose vitamin E as defined as greater than or equal to four hundred IU per day. For the participants in nine of these eleven high-dose studies, vitamin E supplementation resulted in increased death rates with a dose-response effect. That means that the higher the dose of vitamin E, the greater the likelihood that the participant died. The authors concluded that high doses of vitamin E greater than four hundred IU per day should be avoided [238].

- *Antioxidants increased death rates.* Using the data from fourteen randomized trials, supplementation with beta-carotene, vitamin A, vitamin C, or vitamin E failed to protect participants against cancers of the stomach, intestines, liver, and pancreas. In those trials that used the best scientific methods, antioxidant use was linked to higher rates of death for the participants [239].

- *Antioxidants did not prevent cardiovascular disease.* This study evaluated the cardioprotective effect of daily vitamin E, vitamin C, and beta-carotene for 20,536 high-risk individuals. This study did not find any increased death rates associated with antioxidant use, but it also did not discover any protective effect for vascular disease or cancer for antioxidant use over a five-year period [240].

- *Antioxidants did not prevent colon cancer.* This meta-analysis of 17,620 participants who were given vitamin A, vitamin C, vitamin E, beta-carotene, and selenium (alone or in combination) showed no preventive impact on colon cancer [241].

- *Antioxidants did not prevent vision problems.* This multicenter study of 4,629 older adults examined the effect of vitamin C, vitamin E, and beta-carotene on age-related cataract and vision loss. High doses of these antioxidants had no impact on cataract formation or loss of vision [242].

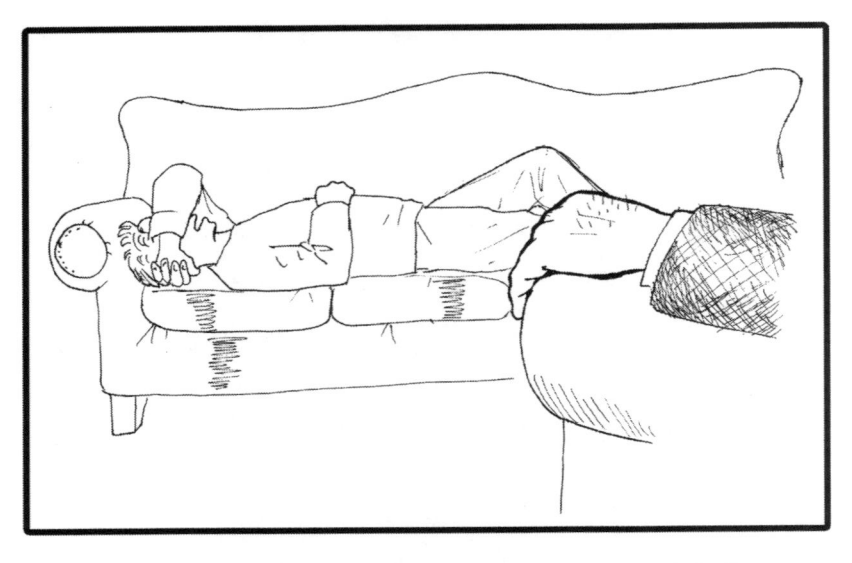

"Doctor, I've decided it's time to end my life."
"Well, you could try vitamin E."

- *Antioxidants did not prevent the common cold.* Do you take high amounts of vitamin C to prevent or treat the common cold? Whether extra vitamin C helps with minor respiratory viruses has been a debated idea for decades. A recent meta-analysis involving 11,306 subjects showed that vitamin C will not prevent a cold; however, taking it when you are sick can reduce the severity and duration of the illness. But don't expect miracles here; the participants studied only exhibited an 8 percent reduction in the duration of the cold as a result of taking vitamin C [243].

Over the years, speculation has increased about the safety of high-dose antioxidants that many nutritional counselors and naturopaths recommend. Let's discuss the largest study in the literature suggesting that antioxidants fail to extend the life-span and may be associated with greater rates of mortality. In 2007, a landmark meta-analysis on antioxidants was conducted that explored the relationship between death rates and antioxidant use [244]. Because antioxidants have been espoused to be the answer for many acute and chronic conditions, the researchers wanted to know if their use helped to increase one's life-span. The results of the study are quite remarkable in that ingestion of high levels of antioxidants (beta-carotene, vitamin A, and vitamin E) were associated with *increased* death rates.

That's right. When single or combined antioxidants were compared to placebo in the results of sixty-eight studies with 232,606 participants, they were associated with increased mortality. This meta-analysis was conducted on 385 pieces of published research and almost a quarter of a million participants. First hearing the results of this study was shocking, but I also have a hard time arguing with the robust correlations documented in this research. Interestingly, the study only investigated the effects for synthetic antioxidants, and so it would be incorrect to generalize these findings to food sources of antioxidants. Also, this study did not study any antioxidants that were applied topically. We can presume that food sources of antioxidants and topical antioxidants continue to be safe.

So, there you have it: a list of powerful clinical studies using thousands of participants that showed either no effect or harmful effects for high-dose antioxidants. When we spend money on supplements, we do so because we also believe that these compounds will improve our overall health. Clearly the efficacy and safety of high-dose antioxidants may be more complicated than we thought. Another consideration in evaluating these studies is that they have huge statistical power. When analyzing data from thousands and thousands of people, the researcher's ability to detect even small relationships between variables increases dramatically. When crunching data from this many participants, even tiny relationships are statistically significant and clinically meaningful. At the end of the day, if there were consistent benefits to be found from antioxidants, these studies would have uncovered them. Unfortunately, they did not.

However, before you throw out your vitamin C, keep in mind that what was demonstrated in these studies was correlation, not causation. We have to be very careful not to assign causation to correlational studies. This means that we have no causal mechanism for how antioxidants led to death in these studies; we only know that high antioxidant use and death happened to occur at the same time. To offer a balanced discussion on this topic, I'll play devil's advocate for a moment. Consider someone who is battling a chronic disease that suddenly gets worse. This person will likely be motivated to try anything to get better. As this person gets closer to death, she may be even more willing to try excessive therapies (like high-dose antioxidants) in an effort to get well. Still, we have to seriously consider the possibility that high-dose antioxidants may be harmful. Let's talk about why in the next section.

Why high-dose antioxidants may not work. We have to wonder why these studies show no benefit from high-dose antioxidants.

I would like to propose a few possibilities. One factor that I would like to note about these studies is that they all used supplementation with antioxidants from pills. If people think they are getting all the nutrients they need from pills, perhaps they are prone to eat fewer natural (and superior) sources of these antioxidants in food. I would be interested to know whether taking supplements actually correlates with lower fruit and vegetable ingestion. Because the antioxidants from food sources may be qualitatively different, and because we know that food sources are more readily absorbed than pills, I have to wonder if we would observe more positive effects if these studies were repeated with food-sourced antioxidants. Additionally, much of the evidence that demonstrates the efficacy of antioxidants has been drawn from rats, not humans. Now, animal models form the core of most preliminary medical research. (Before clinical trials on humans are conducted, efficacy is usually demonstrated on an animal model.) Yet it is still an assumption that the results demonstrated on animal models are generalizable to humans.

As we learn more about vitamins and minerals, it is becoming clear that food sources are more effective than supplement or pill sources. Many nutritional experts have advised caution when taking synthetic antioxidants. First, we don't have a good understanding of whether synthetic versions of antioxidants (compounds made in a chem lab) work the same in the body as naturally occurring compounds. For example, many molecules have a right- and left-oriented version, just like your hands. And like your hands, these right-handed and left-handed molecules function a little differently. We just don't have enough information about these synthetic compounds. Second, you have the absorption problem. Antioxidants from pills just aren't absorbed into the body as well as antioxidants from food. It is estimated that only about 15 percent of the contents of vitamin tablets actually are absorbed into the body. Finally, the studies mentioned point to a great debate about whether high-dose antioxidants are safe to take when a nonfood source is used; supplementation of this type may not even work at all. Although everyone seems to be in agreement that topical antioxidants are risk-free, we need to consider carefully our doses of oral antioxidants as their use may contain risks.

Researchers at the Department for Human Nutrition in Germany [245] have proposed a possible causal explanation for the link between mortality and antioxidant use for humans in the 2007 meta-analysis that we reviewed. Basically, by exposing cells to harsh insults, such as free radicals, cells toughen up and become more prepared to fend off serious disease. The powerhouse of the cell, the mitochondria, are responsible for producing most of the reactive oxygen species inside the cell. As the mitochondria produce more free radicals, this acts as a cellular signaling event. Internal defense mechanisms are activated throughout the organism to help it build stress tolerance and increase life-span. By adding high amounts of antioxidants to the mix, free radicals are reduced, and the reactive oxygen species signaling system is short-circuited. If antioxidants reduce our opportunity to practice fighting off serious incidents, we are then less prepared to deal with illness.

Researchers in the area of internal medicine have given a clear opinion that antioxidants in isolated, pill form are a poor substitution for those found in whole foods. In fact, synthetic sources may be harmful [15]. Furthermore, these authors have stated that only research conducted with whole food-sourced antioxidants has shown any benefit. After reviewing the evidence for and against antioxidants, what do I recommend at the end of the day? I recommend a conservative approach and that you follow the recommended dietary allowances for vitamins, minerals, and macronutrients put out and maintained by the National Agricultural Library, U.S. Department of Agriculture. You can download dietary reference charts online; these dietary recommendations are provided according to age, gender, and special conditions such as pregnancy and lactation. Our discussion about free radicals aside, your body needs adequate amounts of vitamins, minerals, and macronutrients (protein, carbohydrate, and fiber) to biochemically operate and fend off illness. I recommend getting these charts for your personal use and working with your diet to get all of these nutrients from food sources.

To sum up, we are left with a confused picture about whether high-dose antioxidants work and whether they are safe. I can't tell you what is best for you to do, but as for myself, I am letting go of high-priced high-dose antioxidants and am focusing on modifying my diet to improve my food sources of these vital compounds. For example, I bought a juicer, and I feel like juicing my vegetables has been a strong foundation in maintaining my health. About three times a week, I wash, chop, and juice a large French mixing bowl of carrots, cabbage, kale, asparagus, tomatoes, apples, grapefruit, celery, and anything else I can get my hands on. Now that's a lot of veggies. It tastes terrible to get down, but I'm hooked on it because I know I am getting high doses of nutrients in the form that nature intended.

When it comes to vitamins and minerals, it's time to go old school. My grandmother had a career as a nutritionist in a hospital setting. The main focus of her work was designing meals to give people the nutrition they needed from the food the hospital served. She was famous in the hospital for insisting that if you want people to get their nutrition, you have to give them freshly made, nutritious meals that taste good. Fancy that—food should taste good! In the modern world, with both spouses working, schedules are very tight. Under these pressures, it's easy just to reach for the pill bottle and assume that we are getting the nutrition we need. But the research I presented in this chapter indicates that nutrition from synthetic sources just isn't cutting it. Take my grandmother's advice and put the focus of your nutrition on food, not a bottle. If you just cannot make that work, look for a liquid multivitamin to provide basic levels of these nutrients, as liquid sources are more readily absorbable. Finally, if you are not swayed by all of the evidence I presented on the risks associated with high-dose antioxidants (vitamin C, vitamin E, vitamin A, beta-carotene,

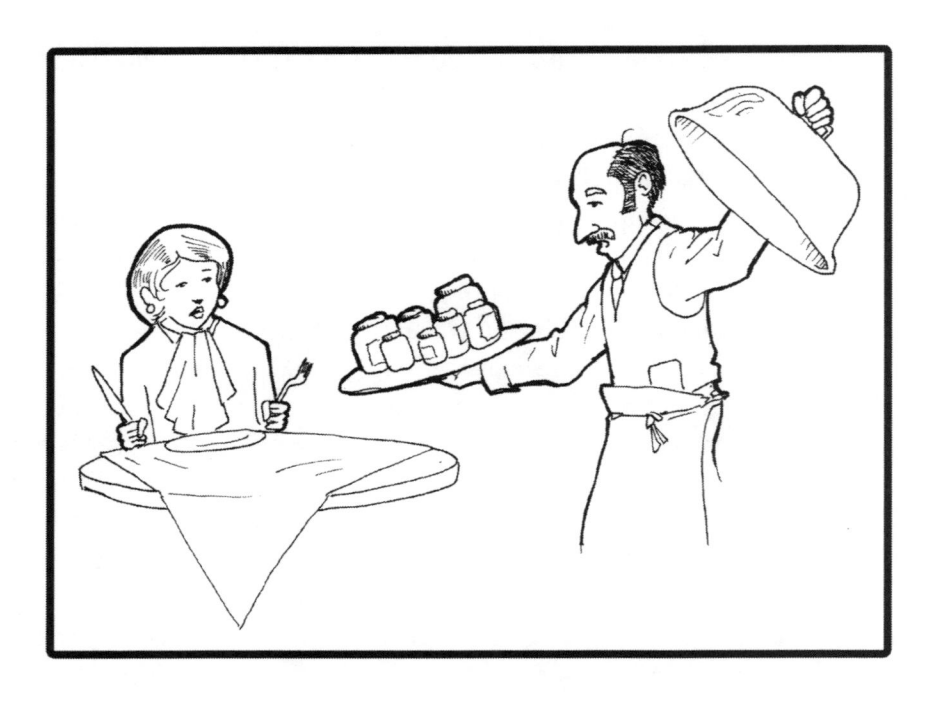

"Your meal, Madame."

etc.), consider using a juicer to get higher doses of nutrients from food sources. By juicing, you can ingest much higher quantities of whole food-sourced nutrients than you would be able to ingest from meals alone.

Let's be frank. People get sick; they get really sick and die. If the medical community had all of the answers, we would all be happily living to the limit of healthy aging (about 120 years old). Neither traditional doctors nor alternative doctors have all the answers. When we get super sick and no one has the answers, we get frightened and will reach for anything. In the midst of our fear, we need to be careful that we don't reach for things that could be harmful to us. I'm taking the money that I used to spend on high-dose antioxidants and putting it toward my 401(k). Maybe antioxidant pills won't give me any extra days, but retiring a little earlier will let me make better use of the days I do have.

Antioxidants and the skin. In 1998, a dermatologist named Peter Pugliese put out a report discussing the importance of antioxidants in maintaining healthy skin [246]. He proposed that all disorders of the skin involve inflammatory components that can be improved by the anti-inflammatory effects of antioxidants. Almost every book and Internet article you read on skin care talks about the importance of topical and oral antioxidants.

What are some antioxidants that are good for skin? Beta-carotene is used to keep skin and the lining of the mucus membranes healthy; it is also believed to assist in skin's repair mechanisms and to increase the natural production of collagen. Increased collagen can reduce the appearance of fine lines and wrinkles because it basically keeps skin "fluffy" and decreases the likelihood that skin will settle into wrinkles. Another antioxidant on our list, selenium, is believed to protect the skin from sun damage and wrinkles when used in topical forms. Finally, vitamin C also helps the body to produce collagen and assists in skin repair.

Most dermatologists agree that topical antioxidants can

help keep the skin age-free. Clinical research has shown that antioxidants do prevent the progression of inflammation in the skin [247]. This study demonstrated that antioxidants modulate inflammation by stopping the migration of chemicals called neutrophils. Many other clinical studies have shown implications of antioxidants in inflammation and the overall health of the skin [248].

Chapter 8

Are Your Feet Getting Heavier?

This chapter discusses clinically proven detoxifying strategies that remove heavy metal pollution from our bodies. Heavy metal contamination of the human body happens when trace amounts of metals become trapped in our tissues. Sources of contamination can include medical implants (like mercury-based dental fillings) as well as food, water, and toiletries that contain small amounts of metal. The list of metals that are harmful to humans includes mercury, nickel, lead, cadmium, chromium, and arsenic [249]. Even though there are only tiny, tiny amounts of these contaminants in our food and water, the body has very poor metabolic strategies for binding these metals and excreting them through the digestive tract or urine. As the years of exposure go by, these trace amounts build up to levels that interfere with basic metabolic processes in the body. As we age, the risk of developing health problems that can be linked back to heavy metal accumulation also increases. Because mercury is one of the most common and poisonous heavy metal contaminants, it will be our focus in this chapter.

Over the last few decades, environmental regulations regarding acceptable levels of heavy metals in food and water have improved in highly industrialized countries. However, much needs to be done to reduce pollution of the environment and how much pollution finds a home in our bodies. Our governments seem to think that there is an acceptable level for heavy metals in our food and water. But I have to wonder

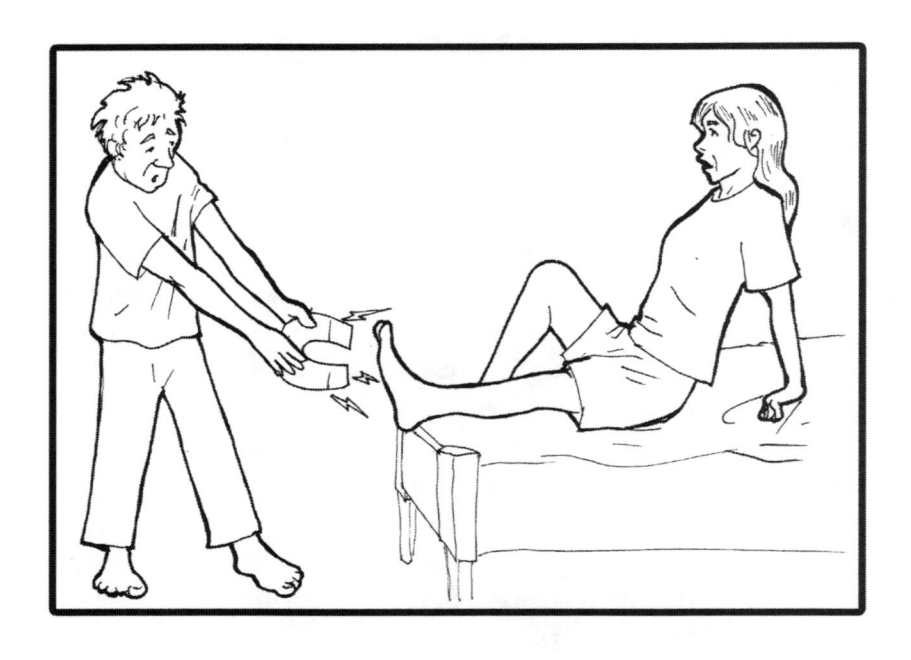

"Darling, I don't think these heavy metals are budging."

whether there really is an acceptable level for compounds that have such catastrophic effects on our health.

Science needs to weigh in on two main questions with regard to heavy metals. First, is there evidence that pollutants from the environment make their way into our bodies? Examining soil samples and geographic rates of lung cancer, a group of researchers in Taiwan demonstrated a relationship between high rates of cancer and heavy metals in the environment [250]. Similar results were found for an abandoned mine in Greece [251]. This research means that we absorb heavy metals through contaminated environments, and this can result in a multitude of health problems. Science has demonstrated that the heavy metals consumed in seafood do find a permanent home in the body. One study measuring the mercury content of women's hair in Iran showed that amounts of mercury were positively related to how much fish the women consumed [252]. These findings have also been replicated on people living in the Czech Republic [253]. Once you eat it, it's there until you treat it.

Now let's deal with the second question that science needs to answer. Is there evidence that heavy metal pollutants increase in our bodies as we age? As we age, our exposure to nonpoint sources of heavy metals increases, simply because of the fact that we have spent more time on a polluted planet. For example, cadmium levels in tumor tissue samples were higher for older people in both smokers *and* nonsmokers [254]. Also, as children with mercury dental amalgams increased in age from eight to eighteen, mercury levels excreted in the urine increased by as much as 52 percent in adulthood [255]. Unfortunately, the amount of measurable mercury in human tissue has increased over the last fifty years to worrying levels [256]. In summary, science has given us clear data indicating that environmental pollutants get trapped in our bodies and also increase in concentration as we age.

Next, you are probably wondering about the biological consequences of age-related heavy metal accumulation. Heavy metal accumulation can also result in vague, systemic symptoms that affect the general quality of life. Using reports from ninety-two patients with mercury poisoning, common clinical symptoms included fatigue, memory problems, headache, dizziness, insomnia, and tremor [257]. Unfortunately, heavy metal contamination can also disrupt the fragile developmental process for young people. Mercury has been implicated in hearing loss in adolescents [258], while heavy metals in general have been implicated in autism [259]. Anecdotally, some autistic children have shown improvements in speech and relational abilities after being treated for heavy metal accumulation. However, the role of heavy metals in the etiology of autism is a much debated topic with various scientific studies coming down on both sides of the argument.

Age-Related Heavy Metal Accumulation

The data implicating heavy metals in human health problems are overwhelming. We can no longer subscribe to a theory of heavy metal poisoning; we must now take it as a scientific fact. But how do heavy metals act to cause these problems? What is the actual mechanism by which these elements cause health problems? Researchers in India have proposed that heavy metals create higher levels of reactive oxygen, or free radicals. These free radicals then circulate through the body, attacking vulnerable systems. Metals also have a strong attraction to proteins and enzymes and can therefore disrupt basic biochemical reactions that the body uses to maintain itself. Finally, metals can affect a variety of chemical messenger compounds, throwing off cellular signaling [260].

Two sources of mercury seem to cause the most concern: mercury amalgam dental fillings and seafood. Let's talk about seafood first. Heavy metals from industrial sources leech into the water table and eventually find their way into our streams, estuaries, and oceans. As with humans, the longer lived a fish is, the greater the likelihood of heavy metal exposure. Also, fish on the higher end of the food chain are also at greater risk for heavy metal accumulation. How does this work? Small plants and floating organisms absorb heavy metals through their cell walls from industrial sources. These creatures are then eaten by slightly larger creatures, such as shrimp. With each meal, the shrimp absorb the lifetime accumulation of heavy metals from the small plants and floating organisms. Smaller fish eat the shrimp, and then larger fish eat the smaller fish. With each meal, a larger fish may be consuming all of the heavy metals accumulated by pounds of small plants. When you eat that fish, you absorb all of the heavy metals accumulated by it during its entire lifetime. Marine biologists now suggest that mercury poisoning may be the reason for the eventual extinction of the whales. A mother whale who nurses her young just happens to be wired to dump massive amounts of her own heavy metal accumulation into the milk for her baby. Across the generations of whales, levels of heavy metals are reaching alarming quantities.

Another major source of concern for human mercury accumulation are mercury dental amalgams, or "silver" fillings. The Scientific Committee on Emerging and Newly Identified Health Risks has issued a report stating that there are no systemic health consequences from dental amalgam. However, a German researcher evaluated the scientific studies used by the committee to write this opinion and found the research to be severely lacking in scientific method [261]. Mutter cited proven autopsy studies that reported two to twelve times more mercury in patients with dental amalgams than in those with no fillings. These autopsy studies found higher mercury content in the brain and kidneys—two organ systems that would seem to correspond to clinical symptom reports for people with this type of poisoning [262]. Finally, Mutter reported that ingested mercury can persist in the brain for decades [261]. One has to wonder about the political and liability considerations that underlie statements that mercury fillings are harmless.

What are mercury amalgams? Mercury dental fillings are 50 percent mercury bound to other compounds [262]. In the past, these types of fillings were believed to be safe because once the mercury was chemically bonded to another atom, it was rendered inert and unable to leave the filling. But think about the metal in your car. When your car was first produced, all of the atoms in the metal were well bound to other atoms. But over time, environmental stress caused these bonds to come apart in the form of rust. What was once a solid piece of metal then began to flake apart over time. Any chemist will tell you that the chemical bonds in any molecule can eventually break down because of environmental stress. This means that what started as bound, inert mercury can turn into unbound mercury gas that is absorbed into the body as time goes by. If you have ever broken an old mercury-filled thermometer, you may remember that the mercury very quickly evaporated into a gas. It is astounding to me that the dental community settled on such as unstable element on which to base its cavity-filling technology. One enlightened dentist told me that people will look back at mercury fillings as the greatest health crisis of the century.

We know that mercury vapor is continuously emitted from aging mercury amalgams. Researchers estimate that one mercury amalgam filled tooth emits about one-half to one microgram per day of mercury vapor, which is then absorbed into the body. Using exposure levels put out by the U.S. Environmental Protection Agency and the number of teeth filled with mercury by the average American, approximately seventy million Americans would exceed acceptable levels of mercury exposure during the first decade of the twenty-first century [263]. Other researchers have also documented dental amalgams as a significant culprit in mercury accumulation as measured by mercury in the urine; more mercury fillings were correlated with higher levels of biochemical markers of mercury burden in the urine [264]. Like whale mothers, human mothers also pass on their accumulated mercury to their offspring in breast milk. In this study, mercury levels in the breast milk of new mothers were correlated with the number of amalgam fillings. For participants, exposure to mercury from breast milk would be high enough to affect infant health, according to recommendations by the World Health Organization [265]. When my holistic physician saw the number of mercury fillings I had, he immediately showed me a video of a mercury filling that captured the escaping mercury vapor. You can easily view one of these videos with a simple Internet search. The mercury gas just pours off of old dental amalgam.

The body needs help to get those heavy metals back out again. Because so many of us may have been exposed to heavy metal accumulation, I'd like to review the current options for heavy metal detoxification. A good detoxification program administered by your holistic physician will begin with a simple screening test using a sample of hair. On the basis of the number of mercury amalgam fillings in my mouth (ten), I was immediately sent to have this test. If you have a history of mercury fillings or high seafood consumption, consider having this simple and noninvasive test for heavy metal accumulation. The hair sample is sent to a lab, where it is analyzed for heavy metal content; your results are then interpreted by your doctor. My results were off the chart, and I was immediately referred for an aggressive heavy metal detoxification program. Depending on the results of your hair sample test, your doctor may recommend an individualized approach to your detoxification. Currently the options include nutritional supplements for mild exposure and aggressive chelation therapy for severe cases. The FDA has not approved any over-the-counter products for the chelation of heavy metals. As with most things in the alternative health world, there is a great deal of controversy surrounding treatments for heavy metal accumulation. Let's look at some of the research on these options so you can have an informed conversation with your doctor.

Chlorella. Chlorella vulgaris is a single-celled algae with a particular affinity for absorbing heavy metals through its cell walls. In fact, this algae is so powerful in attracting and binding heavy metals that it is used at environmental cleanup sites to

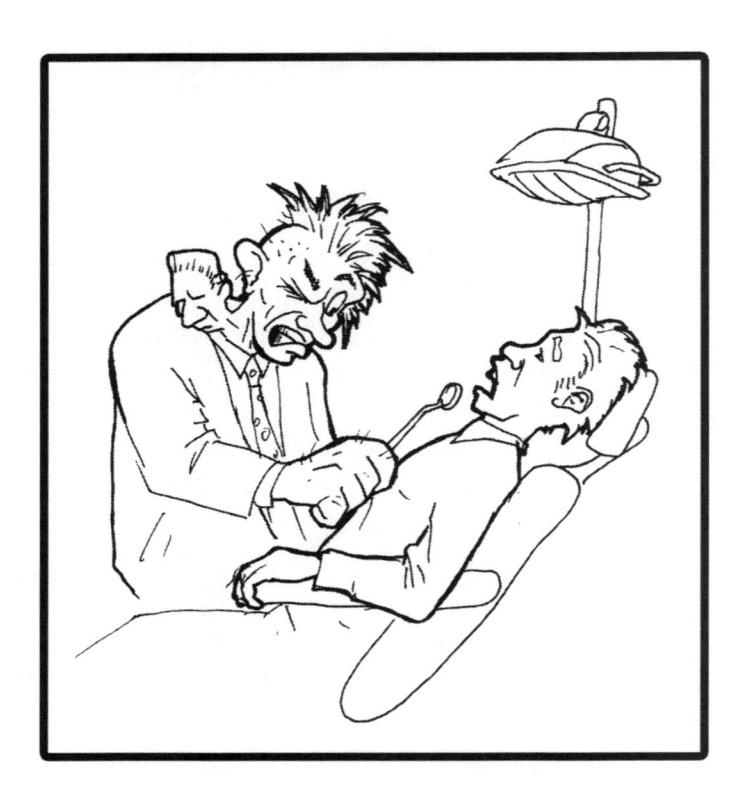

"Dr. Dentist, I don't think I want mercury in my body."
"They're fine! I have 12!"

remove heavy metal contamination [266,267]. Your doctor may begin an extensive heavy metal detox program with chlorella or recommend supplementation with this algae for mild cases of accumulation. Talk to your doctor if daily supplementation with chlorella is right for you.

Animal model studies have demonstrated efficacy for this algae in repairing damage due to heavy metals [268]. In this study, chlorella was able to repair lead-induced effects to bone marrow and cytokine production in mice. In another mouse study, oral supplementation with chlorella prevented lead from being absorbed by the gastrointestinal tract [269]. This is big news, because many of us acquire much of our heavy metal accumulation through contaminated food sources. If chlorella can help deter the body from absorbing heavy metals from food sources through the digestive tract, then daily supplementation could also help us to prevent age-related environmental exposure through food. Also in the study, chlorella promoted the excretion of lead in the feces and is another indicator that chlorella helps the body keep lead moving rather than absorbing it deeper into the tissues. What about chlorella for other heavy metals? In the body, mercury can combine with other compounds to produce methylmercury—a highly toxic molecule. When mice were administered methylmercury and then provided with a continuous intake of chlorella, they were able to increase their excretion of methylmercury. This enhanced excretion eventually led to a measurable decrease in elemental mercury in the tissues [270].

Chelation therapy. Chelation therapy is the use of intravenous, intramuscular, or oral compounds to bind heavy metals in a form that can be excreted by the body in the urine and feces. Again, the FDA has not approved any chelating agents for over-the-counter use, but a number of clinical studies have demonstrated both safety and symptom improvement for physician-administered chelation agents with respect to heavy metal poisoning. The two most well-accepted chelating agents are dimercapto-propane sulfonate (DMPS) and dimercaptosuccinic acid (DMSA) [260]. Your doctor will examine your individual heavy metal profile from your testing and choose the right chelation agent for you; the different agents have different affinities for specific metals. In a study of fifty-eight children who received a daily course of DMSA, no adverse effects from the therapy were observed [271]. However, some authors have discussed side effects from using these agents [260].

Are chelating agents successful in reducing the heavy metal load in the body? Clinical studies suggest that they are effective. In one study of ninety-two patients with mercury poisoning, symptoms were gradually reduced over time. Interestingly, symptoms were alleviated at different rates in different body systems, with cardiovascular symptoms resolving in two weeks and neurological symptoms resolving in three months [257]. DMPS and DMSA have also been administered to mercury-poisoned pregnant rats to demonstrate that mercury ions were reduced in the tissue of the mother and the fetus as a result of treatment [272]. Another clinical study was conducted on patients with dental amalgams to show that those with mercury fillings exhibit greater mercury levels; patients with fillings excreted more mercury in the urine in response to DMPS than patients with no fillings [273]. Finally, once dental amalgams were removed from the mouth, patients reported a significant improvement in mercury-related symptoms following treatment with DMPS. The most alarming symptoms reported by patients in this study were fatigue, backache, and neurological problems; all symptoms demonstrated improvement on average, with 78 percent of patients reporting satisfaction with their treatment [274].

Some authors have suggested that severe heavy metal poisoning must be managed long term by periodic treatments with chelating agents. A few weeks after completing treatment with DMSA, the blood concentration levels of lead returned to approximately 58 percent of the value before treatment [271]. In another study, DMPS was shown to reduce blood levels of mercury for a period of time, and this transitory reduction in serum levels is associated with a reduction in mercury-related symptoms. The authors recommended repeated treatment with DMPS to manage serum mercury levels [275]. These findings suggest that chelating agents target their action on blood levels of heavy metals. Over time, heavy metals can leech back into the bloodstream from contaminated tissues, thus necessitating a repeat of the treatment to keep circulating levels of metals below clinical levels. Talk to your doctor about what kind of maintenance therapy is recommended based on your individual profile of heavy metal contamination. Finally, the research is mixed on whether adding antioxidant supplements to chelation therapy contributes to the binding and excretion of heavy metals [276].

Chapter 9

Plant an Inner Garden

In this chapter, we talk about digestive health and how problems in the digestive tract can contribute to premature health concerns. Let's talk about the pipes in your house as a metaphor for understanding how the digestive tract ages. If you have ever seen the inside of old pipes, it can be quite alarming. Opening up the pipe that runs out of your kitchen sink into your garbage disposal will reveal a slimy layer of rotting food. This layer of rotting garbage provides an apartment complex for wandering bacteria and fungi just looking for a permanent home and steady food supply. This is going to be a hard image to digest (sorry, couldn't resist that pun), but the line out from your kitchen sink works exactly the same as your digestive tract. When your pipes were first placed in your kitchen, they were uncorroded and gleaming. But over time, food, bacteria, and fungi gradually found a foothold in the grooves of the metal invisible to the naked eye. It's the same with your intestines, the "line out" from your stomach. Over the years, opportunistic bacteria and fungi are able to capitalize on every opportunity to gain a foothold on your intestinal walls. What was once pristine tissue may now be a mess of invasive organisms and hardened stool that the body can't get rid of. In addition, the alternative health community generally regards fecal accumulation as a by-product of the aging process. With age, the muscles in the abdomen become less effective at moving waste out of the body. When the body can't rid itself of all its stool, the colon simply

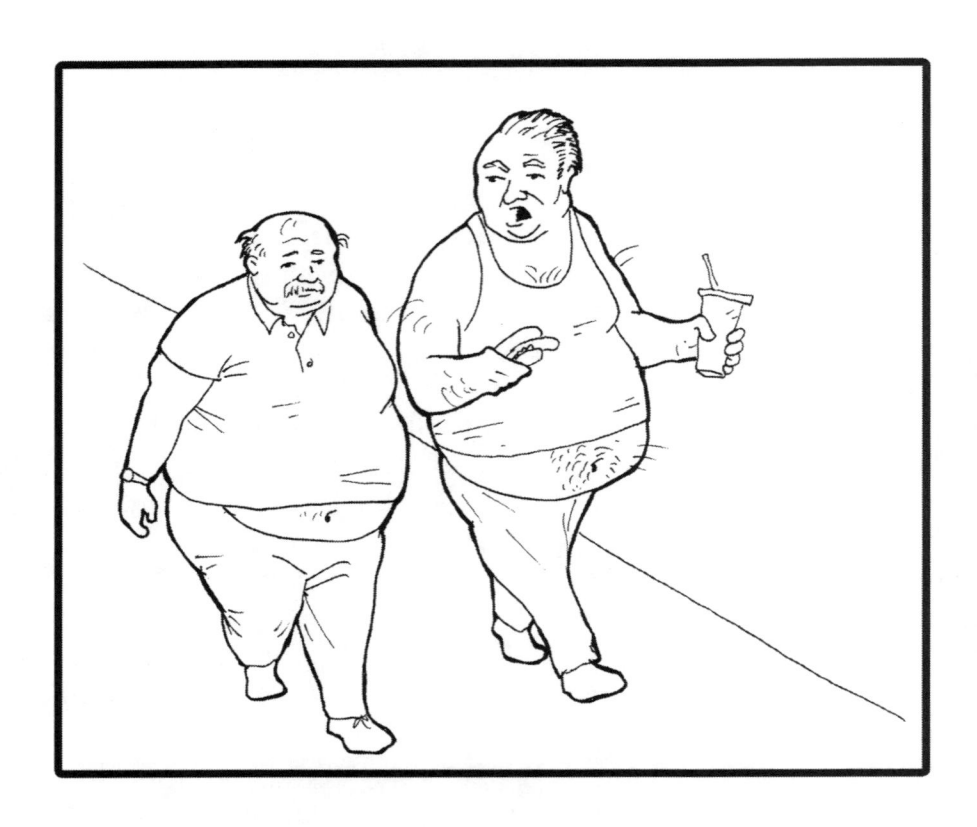

"I don't understand why all women can't look like supermodels."

expands to accommodate it, resulting in weight gain and an increase in gut size.

As we age, the beneficial bacteria in the gut can become out of balance. With each round of antibiotics we take, we risk developing resistant bugs and disturbing the fragile balance of probiotic bacteria in the digestive tract. Here is another metaphor to help you understand how the tissue of your digestive tract works. The tissue through which food moves and is processed is porous; it has little holes in it like the screen in your window. Why? Because nutrients and energy sources need to pass out of your food and get absorbed into the body. If this tissue were completely solid, you would die from lack of nutrient absorption. In a normal, healthy colon, the holes in the "screen" are teeming with friendly bacteria. Probiotics fill in these holes in the tissue and help to form a semisolid shield between waste and the rest of the body. When the friendly bacteria in the gut get depleted from antibiotic use and food pollutants, the holes in your "screen" become larger than they should be. Instead of only allowing nutrients to pass, the tissues of the colon now allow toxins from waste and endotoxins from unfriendly bacteria to enter the bloodstream. Your body treats these invasive chemicals like invaders and triggers inflammatory processes throughout the body. With chronic exposure, the immune system becomes confused and fatigued. This person's body now becomes less able to fight off actual invaders because it's too busy attacking the wastes that have entered the body. With the immune system in a constant state of alarm, it may begin to attack normal, healthy tissue by mistake and develop into an autoimmune disorder of the colon [277].

This problem of heightened gut permeability is called *leaky gut syndrome* by both the scientific and alternative healing communities. If you can tolerate an even more graphic image, think about what recently left your body in the bathroom; now imagine that stuff leaking through the intestinal wall and back into the body. When the permeability of the digestive tract is higher than it should be, it can result in a variety of conditions, including allergies, metabolic disturbances, or cardiovascular problems [278]. Gut permeability is also thought to be one of the underlying factors in digestive disorders like irritable bowel syndrome [279]. Has science been able to demonstrate a relationship between the size of the holes in the intestines and digestive disorders? I'm glad you asked. Medical researchers looked at the amount of intestinal permeability for two major digestive disorders: irritable bowel syndrome and ulcerative colitis. For both groups of patients with these disorders, the permeability of the colon was significantly greater as compared to healthy volunteers [280].

Not only are digestive disorders implicated with leaky gut syndrome but other modern medical mysteries may also be explained. One such example is chronic fatigue syndrome (CFS). There is now the scientific suggestion that one of the contributing factors to CFS is the movement of bacterial endotoxins through the gut wall and into the bloodstream. These toxins contribute to the malaise and fatigue that characterize CFS. In one remarkable case study with a thirteen-year-old girl with CFS, treatment with a diet targeted to heal the gut stopped the movement of endotoxins across the gut wall. When her serum IgM in response to bacterial endotoxin normalized on the new diet, her CFS symptoms were cured completely [281].

In this chapter, we talk about one high-powered probiotic and two nutritional supplements that can help to heal the gut. However, one of the most important supplements to use in healing the bowel is the master anti-aging supplement that we have covered throughout this book. Douglas Wyatt, the director for research at the Center for Nutritional Research and considered by many to be the father of colostrum, described colostrum as the most important supplement that you can take to heal leaky gut syndrome. (For more information on how colostrum can help heal the bowel and the body overall, be sure to check out information from the Center for Nutritional

Research online.) How does colostrum heal the bowel? It delivers immunoglobulins to defeat invasive bacteria and growth factors that help restore the connection between cells in the intestinal lining.

A medical science writer named Shawn Green [81] has talked about the importance of colostrum in healing the symptoms of leaky gut. He offers the syndrome of HIV as a model for understanding how the gut becomes too permeable:

> The gut in chronic HIV-1-infected individuals appears to be reminiscent of newborn calves. Calves are born with a highly immature mucosal immune system and "leaky gut" which, if not immediately corrected, results in death due to infection and associated systemic immune activation. However, the cow's first milk rescues her calves from harmful gut microbes with a uniquely complex cocktail enriched with neutralizing polyclonal antibodies, cytokine tissue repair factors, and immune enhancing probiotics, such as Lactobacillus species. Regular consumption of biologically active bovine colostrum has been known for years to promote the development of infantile gut-associated lymphoid tissue and enhance CD4 levels, while suppressing CD8 and inflammatory bowel disease (IBD), including ulcerative colitis and Crohn's Disease.

Now, what is he really saying? Here he gives a more clinical description of what we discussed at the beginning of this chapter. When the gut is infected with bacteria, endotoxins from the bacteria are absorbed through the intestinal wall and into the body. When many bacteria are present and are being killed by the immune system, too many lipopolysaccharides (endotoxins) from the cell walls of gram-negative bacteria are dumped into the body. Essentially, these toxins overwhelm the liver and lymph drainage systems. This results in endotoxin contamination, a huge source of inflammation in the body. If the inflammation response is severe, the patient can go into septic shock. Just remember that high bacterial death = endotoxin = bad.

If the intestinal wall is not properly formed yet (as in the case of the human infant) or is not properly protected by the immune system (as in the case of the HIV+ patient), it becomes more easy for endotoxins to pass from the digestive tract and into the body, where they can cause inflammation and other problems [282]. Colostrum can help the HIV patient to recover gut immunity and become more resistant to the problem called microbial endotoxin translocation [81]. In fact, studies have shown that colostrum alleviates diarrhea for the HIV+ patient and results in increases in peripheral blood CD4 T cells and body weight [283]. Colostrum can offer new hope for anyone suffering from increased gut permeability. Because oral administration of colostrum delivers it right to the intestinal wall, the digestive distressed person can receive colostrum right where it is needed.

Rebalancing the Digestive Tract

This chapter outlines three additional supplements that may be used to restore the balance of bacteria and fungi in the gut to a more youthful, healthy state. Talk to your doctor to find out if each one is right for you. If so, your doctor will likely recommend a six-month protocol of this combination therapy that reduces anaerobic and opportunistic organisms while replenishing with colon-friendly probiotics. Your inner garden will be resilient and disease resistant. In addition, restoring the levels of friendly bacteria to normal helps prevent age-related weight gain. Think of beneficial bacteria like tiny rollers that keep your digested food moving along at the right speed. Without these rollers, it's easier for waste to get stuck and develop into hard stools that your body can't eliminate. As food spends more time in the colon than it should, you absorb higher amounts of calories. The following protocol is designed to bring the flora of the digestive tract back into balance and to restore the amount of space between all the cells in the tissue of the gut to more healthy levels.

VSL #3. As we age, we develop a higher risk for probiotic imbalance in the gut because of greater exposure to medications and environmental pollutants. If you have had more than a handful of antibiotic courses across your lifetime, chances are that the friendly bacteria in your digestive tract are not as prevalent as they should be. Some aggressive alternative health providers have proposed that any administration of antibiotics leaves antibiotic-resistant organisms in the body. With repeated antibiotic use, these organisms can build up and become dominant. Also, when antibiotics kill the bacteria in your gut, space opens up for preexisting yeast and fungi to develop beyond healthy levels. Adequate supplementation with the right probiotic will eventually push out invasive candida and other fungi. Remember, your body wants to heal; health is its natural state. When we restore the correct probiotic strains to the digestive tract, studies have confirmed improvement in inflammatory markers, improvement in the stability of the gut barrier, and a reduction in the hypersensitivity of the digestive tissue [279].

The most powerful probiotic on the market is called VSL #3. It is also the probiotic product with the most clinical evidence supporting its use for repopulating the digestive tract with friendly bacteria. Although you can purchase it from your local pharmacy or through the mail without a prescription, VSL #3 is considered a medical food and should be used only under the supervision of a licensed medical provider. This is because the probiotic dose is so high as compared to other products. VSL #3 was created for the dietary management of IBDs, but it can also be used to help people with systemic candida and bacterial imbalance in the gut. What follows is information on the clinical effectiveness of VSL #3 so that you can have an informed conversation with your doctor about whether this brand of probiotic is right for you and how much to take. After being on extended antibiotic therapy for Lyme, my gastroenterologist told me that I had destroyed the natural balance of bacteria and yeasts in my gut. She recommended two packets of VSL #3 a day (about nine hundred billion organisms) for six months to repopulate my digestive tract. Be informed that grocery-store probiotics of one million organisms in a serving are not even worth taking because the numbers of colony-forming units are so small. Consider five billion organisms a day as the minimum effective dose you can take of over-the-counter probiotics.

VSL #3 is made with eight strains of bacteria that occur naturally in the digestive tract:

- *Bifidobacterium breve*
- *Bifidobacterium longum*
- *Bifidobacterium infantis*
- *Lactobacillus acidophilus*
- *Lactobacillus plantarum*
- *Lactobacillus paracasei*
- *Lactobacillus bulgaricus*
- *Streptococcus thermophiles*

Many studies have been conducted showing the positive effects of VSL #3 on many bowel conditions. This medical food is used to treat inflammatory conditions of the bowel, such as ulcerative colitis, and can help prevent recurrences for patients with ulcerative colitis in remission. Oral administration of VSL #3 has also been shown to prevent the development of bacterial pouchitis for patients who have been given a surgical pouch [284]. After eight weeks of treatment with 3,600 billion colony-forming units (CFU) per day, VSL #3 was shown to reduce relapse in ulcerative colitis patients and overall ulcerative colitis symptoms [285,286].

Not only does VSL #3 treat severe IBDs, it has also been shown to help with everyday digestive problems like diarrhea and ulcers. A study was conducted with hospital patients who were given antibiotics and either nine hundred billion CFU of VSL #3 a day or placebo. The VSL #3 group took the therapy during antibiotic use and for one week after the conclusion of antibiotics. None of the VSL #3 treated patients developed antibiotic-associated diarrhea, whereas 11 percent of the placebo group became symptomatic [287]. VSL #3 has also been shown to prevent severe diarrhea after chemotherapy and has been recommended for clinical use by cancer patients [288]. Your stomach also needs to maintain a sufficient complement of friendly bacteria to stay healthy. Finally, VSL #3 has been shown to enhance stomach ulcer healing in a dose-response curve in an animal model. That means that faster healing was achieved with higher amounts of the probiotic [289].

Garlic. Garlic is another supplement that is used by holistic practitioners to rebalance the gut flora. The active ingredient of garlic, allicin, is a natural antibiotic and fungicide. Allicin is the compound that the garlic plant uses to kill pests that attack it. It turns out that allicin works for us, too. Garlic has been used across the world for centuries to manage health before antibiotics and antifungals were available. Garlic is a potent anti-inflammatory agent [290] and seems to be good for a remarkable number of health ailments [291]. Garlic has been scientifically studied and demonstrated efficacy for high blood pressure, high cholesterol, and glycemia. It has also demonstrated clinical activity against bacteria, viruses, fungi, and parasites. When used for longer than two months, garlic can reduce low-density cholesterol by an average of nine milligrams per deciliter for those with high cholesterol [292,293]. When you purchase a garlic product, look for a high allicin content and for garlic that has been freeze-dried rather than heated during processing.

How does garlic help to rebalance what lives in the digestive tract? First, garlic helps beneficial bacteria grow and proliferate in the gut. In this study, garlic powder showed a bactericidal effect against invasive gut bacteria such as *Clostridium nexile*, while friendly gut bacteria, such as lactobacilli, exhibited a resistance to garlic [294]. This means that garlic can help balance the gut by suppressive invasive bacteria while allowing probiotics to flourish. Using a simulated stomach environment, garlic was shown to be effective against *Heliocobacter pylori*. *H. pylori* is a gram-negative bacteria that infects the stomach and can cause chronic gastritis and ulcers. In this study, garlic was shown to rapidly kill *H. pylori* in artificial gastric juice [295]. But how does garlic kill bacteria? Using a very special microscope (beyond our description here), researchers were able to confirm cell injury and death from exposure to garlic. Garlic damages the cell walls of bacterial enemies. By increasing the amounts of organosulfur compounds (like allicin) in the sample, the researchers were able to demonstrate greater killing power [296].

The health of your gut can also be compromised by an overgrowth of fungi including, but not limited to, systemic candida. When we kill too many probiotics, fungal invaders just move right in. Not only does garlic help to rebalance the bacterial complement of the gut but it also kills fungi. Garlic has been shown to be a potent fungicide to a variety of fungal pathogens [297,298]. Furthermore, the addition of allicin to prescription fungicides was shown to increase their effectiveness for *Saccharomyces cerevisiae* by causing structural damage to the yeast vacuole [299].

Finally, keep in mind that garlic is a blood thinner, like aspirin. Blood thinners interfere with how well your platelets stick together. Therefore garlic cannot be used during pregnancy or when getting a surgical procedure. Speak to your doctor about whether you have a medical condition that would restrict you from taking garlic as a nutritional supplement to balance the bowel. Garlic can also interfere with the activity of certain medications.

Olive leaf. The next supplement to consider adding to your digestive balancing protocol is the leaf of the olive tree, *Olea europaea*. Across history, olive leaf has been used to manage a variety of disorders from rheumatism to vascular disease. Studies using an animal model have shown olive leaf to have potent anti-inflammatory properties [300]. It has also demonstrated efficacy against a variety of invasive organisms, including gram-negative bacteria, gram-positive bacteria, and fungi [301]. This neutraceutical has shown combined activity against bacteria and fungi that specifically target the respiratory and intestinal tracts [302].

Where the digestive tract is concerned, olive leaf has been shown to selectively regulate stomach bacteria [303]. In this study, olive leaf was tested on a variety of microorganisms to determine which were sensitive to its action. The authors concluded that olive leaf was not a broad-spectrum antimicrobial but instead was only active against those bacteria that were likely to invade the digestive tract. This work indicates that olive leaf can help regulate the diversity of bacteria in the gut and select against invasive bacteria such as *H. pylori* and *Campylobacter jejuni*. Other research has shown that olive leaf can help regulate other microorganisms that are capable of overpopulating the digestive tract: *E. coli* and *C. albicans* [304]. Finally, another study looked at food-borne pathogens that have a high likelihood of invading the digestive tissue when we ingest them. Olive leaf was shown to kill *E. coli, Salmonella enterica, Staphylococcus aureus,* and *Listeria monocytogenes* [305].

With all of this evidence in hand, we can conclude that supplementation with olive leaf has a high likelihood of suppressing invasive microorganisms in the digestive tract. With a little bit of help from olive leaf, your immune system may be better able to prevent these organisms from gaining a foothold in your system. By combining VSL #3, freeze-dried garlic, olive leaf, and colostrum under a doctor's supervision, the levels of invasive microorganisms will go down, while levels of probiotics will increase to their predisease state.

Chapter 10

What Your Skin Needs Most

SKIN IS THE ORGAN OF the body that first shows signs of aging. You probably don't think of skin as being important to the overall function of the body, but skin is one of your most important organs because it interfaces with the environment and forms a barrier to pathogens. Skin provides insulation, helps regulate temperature, gives us our sense of touch, and makes vitamin D. We even breathe through the skin, as oxygen and nitrogen can diffuse through the skin in small amounts. In this chapter, we talk about how skin ages and discuss a few topical treatments to maintain your youthful glow.

The Science of Healthy Skin

The skin is made of three layers: the epidermis, the dermis, and the underlying fat layer. With the aging process, the epidermis becomes thicker (as a defense against sun, pollution, etc.), whereas the dermis and fat layer become thinner. The dermis layer is extremely important to skin health as it consists mainly of collagen and elastin fibers. These fibers form a network that stretches and gives support to the epidermis layer. How does skin change as we age? These collagen and elastin fibers break down over time, *and* the production of new collagen and elastin fibers slows down. When skin loses its spring, folds settle into wrinkles rather than stretching back to a smooth surface [306]. It becomes vulnerable to age spots, wrinkles, dryness, and loosening because of loss of fat under the surface.

Research has determined that there are two distinct factors that affect aging: internal and external [307]. Intrinsic aging has to do with natural aging processes. This type of aging is governed by the content of DNA inherited from parents, and it affects which extrinsic factors can affect skin to the greatest degree [308]. If you didn't choose your parents very well, then your skin may be prematurely aging. Our DNA determines when the production of collagen slows down and how quickly old skin cells slough off to make room for new, healthier cells. Young people exhibit a dense network of collagen fibers; these fibers become thicker and less well distributed as we get older [309]. As these changes happen, our skin loses its ability to be elastic and to snap back into place. You can think of the collagen like a rubber band. When you first start using a rubber band, it's got a lot of tension and "snap-back-ed-ness." The more you use the rubber band and stretch it over time, the more snap-back-ed-ness it loses, becoming limp and sometimes brittle. With the decline of collagen, your skin becomes limp and brittle like an overused rubber band. When you stretch it, it no longer has as much ability to snap back into place. Unfortunately, there isn't a whole lot you can do to change your DNA.

The second type of skin aging is extrinsic aging. These are external factors that act on the skin to accelerate the aging process. One of the major factors in aging skin is the effect of ultraviolet light on skin repair mechanisms. A few minutes of sun exposure a day can add up to significant negative consequences for your skin over time. Some sun-related changes to the skin can include age spots, freckles, spider veins on the face, fine wrinkles, and leathery texture. Dermatologists refer to this type of aging as *photoaging* [310]. Additionally, cigarette smoking has been directly linked to aging skin: wrinkles increase with the number of cigarettes and the number of years the person has smoked [311,312].

If you have a fair complexion, you are more likely to show the effects of photoaging. Using a daily sunscreen (SPF 15 or above) is absolutely essential for those with fair skin. But even if you have a darker skin type, a daily sunscreen is also necessary. The proof is in—sunblocks do protect us against the UV damage that leads to premature aging. In one study using controlled radiation exposure to simulate sunlight, a number of skin changes were observed in response to exposure [313]. First, the radiated skin exhibited melanization, that is, an increase in the melanin of the skin. Melanin is the dark colored stuff that your skin metabolizes to block sun exposure. (We are just talking about a tan here, folks.) Second, the exposed skin showed changes in thickness. Sun exposure is associated with skin thickening that can lead to a "leathery" look. Last, some biochemical changes were also observed on the skin's elastin fibers using immunofluorescence techniques. When subjects used a sunblock cream with photoprotection properties against UV-A and UV-B radiation, *none* of these effects were observed.

Research has shown that sun-protective behavior differs for men and women and that women are at a greater risk for photoaging because of the ways they choose to protect themselves from the sun [314]. Regardless, a study was conducted at a beach in Belgium to assess skin protection behavior at two time points, one decade apart. Skin aging and skin cancer risk awareness stayed the same over time, with women being more aware than men. However, risk awareness for sunburn did increase over time for women, indicating that educational efforts about damage from sunburn have been effective. The researchers also looked at sun protection strategies. For women, sunscreen was the most popular protection strategy over time, whereas men preferred protective clothing like hats and shirts. It is also likely that gender-based expectations for appearance cause women to prefer sunscreen instead of physical barriers. When we are at the beach, women are supposed to take it off, right? Unfortunately for women, clothing offers a much better protection against photoaging than sunscreens. Once again, women are in double jeopardy—gender role expectations tell us that we need to show our bodies at the beach. But even with sunscreen on board, we are at a higher risk for photoaging than men who choose a protective shirt. After women damage their skin from sun exposure, they are then penalized for aged skin to a greater degree than men. Ladies, it's time to let go of gender-based expectations for showing skin at the beach. Put on a shirt and buy a sexy hat.

Turning Your Everyday Moisturizer into a Fancy Wrinkle Cream

This first strategy for returning skin to a healthy state uses the master anti-aging supplement as a topical treatment to deliver all the healing factors in colostrum right to the skin. By using colostrum as a cosmeceutical, you can deliver epidermal growth factors (the body's own repair messengers) right to the skin. There are many colostrum creams on the market you can purchase for your skin that cost around $20. When I recently conducted market research on cosmetic wrinkle creams, I found that wrinkle creams can run from $50 to as much as $175 a bottle. Colostrum cream is significantly less expensive than most wrinkle creams on the market and does the same job. I even found a few highly expensive wrinkle creams made with epidermal growth factor—the same stuff in colostrum that heals your skin. By choosing one of these products, you are relying on the scientists to make the right decisions about how to formulate and deliver the correct type and amount of growth factors to your skin. Why spend all this money and put your trust in a capitalistic enterprise to deliver the same thing that you can get naturally from colostrum? Mother Nature has perfected the type and amount of growth factors that your body needs to heal the skin. If I was a betting person, I'd be putting my money on Mother Nature. Because I am a spending person, I'm buying colostrum.

Consider trying one of these colostrum creams for your skin by applying it twice a day. You can also turn your everyday moisturizer into a fancy, epidermal growth factor–filled cream by mixing it with colostrum. To do this, purchase a moisturizer that comes in a wide-mouth canister that will allow you to scoop some out. Also purchase a second canister to hold your new beauty cream. Using a clean bowl, begin by emptying all of the moisturizer into it. By eye-balling the empty canister, figure out about how much a quarter of the canister would be. Then add one quarter of this volume of colostrum. You can accomplish this by opening individual capsules of colostrum (pull apart the two halves of the clear capsule covering) or spooning loose colostrum powder into the bowl. Using a clean, dry spoon, blend your mixture well. Colostrum tends to have a grainy texture; be sure to continue stirring until your mixture becomes smooth and thick. Now, divide your mixture between the two containers and apply two times a day to freshly washed skin. You just made your own epidermal growth factor wrinkle cream. Give yourself a pat on the back.

The Master Mask

In previous chapters, we discussed how oral supplementation and topical applications of colostrum can truly do a miracle repair job on your skin. For this technique, we are going to prepare a colostrum mask for the skin. Making a mask from colostrum will ensure that all the skin repair compounds are delivered right to the skin. Even if you take colostrum orally to improve skin and general health, you should still consider this weekly mask technique.

As a base for this mask, we are going to use yogurt. I first learned about using yogurt as a skin treatment from one of my Indian friends while living in California. Indian women have a long tradition of using yogurt as a skin remedy. Because yogurt figures so strongly in the Indian diet, many Indian homemakers prepare their own yogurt to go with their meals. As fresh, live-culture yogurt was readily available, Indian women began using it as a skin treatment. Making fresh yogurt works a lot like San Franciscan sourdough. Sourdough uses live yeast cultures to make the dough rise and acid-producing bacteria to give it that distinctive sour flavor. When the yeast and bacteria have finished their work, a starter ball is set aside to colonize the next batch of flour. When yogurt is made from fresh milk, you seed the milk mixture with live yogurt bacteria that turn the milk into a creamy solid. When the bacteria have finished their work, a small portion of the mixture is set aside and kept alive to colonize the next batch of milk.

I'm sure that very few of you have tasted fresh yogurt. My invitation to my Indian friend's household was the first time that I had ever tasted it. I can tell you that it is absolutely amazing — and so much tastier than the yogurt I grew up with from the grocery store. It's kind of like the difference between a fresh tomato and a canned one. If you are feeling adventurous, or looking for a fun activity to do with the children, you can make your own yogurt using a store-bought starter with live active cultures. There are plenty of recipes online for how to make your own fresh yogurt. However, store-bought yogurt will work for this mask technique as long as it includes live yogurt cultures.

Place about a quarter cup of yogurt into a clean bowl. Next, you are going to add some powdered colostrum. If you have colostrum capsules on hand, empty about ten of them into your yogurt mixture. If you bought the powered form of colostrum, put a heaping tablespoon into your mixture. Stir well and apply the mixture to freshly washed skin. Once the yogurt–colostrum mask has dried on your skin, wash it off. To gauge the impact of this mask on the quality of your skin, repeat the procedure once a week for six weeks. If you really want to go to town with your colostrum mask, add the colostrum to the probiotic mask described in the next section.

The Probiotic Face Mask

The next strategy that I would like to share with you for maintaining great-looking skin is a probiotic face mask. If you are at all connected to the world of holistic medicine and alternative health, you know about the importance of probiotics. When we take antibiotics for an illness, they kill both the good bacteria and the bad bacteria. Your body needs to maintain a certain level of good bacteria to help it prevent and fight off disease. With repeated courses of antibiotics, the levels of probiotics can become depleted, making us even more vulnerable to infection. In fact, experts say that we need a couple of pounds of friendly bacteria in the body to maintain good health. When you consider how much one bacterium would weigh, that's a lot of probiotics!

Like the stomach and nose, the skin is open to invasion by unfriendly bacteria. These bacteria can irritate the skin, get stuck in pores, and cause acne. Your skin is also populated by friendly bacteria. These friendly bacteria live on the skin, and in pores, and form a physical barrier that deters infection. But like other parts of the body, the surface of the skin can become depleted of friendly bacteria. Periodically, you need to replenish the diversity of the friendly bacteria on the skin.

Using this technique, you will mix a probiotic mask from simple ingredients you can find at your local health food store. To get those good bacteria back into pores, you want to buy some yogurt from the store that has live, active cultures of bacteria. I prefer to use plain yogurt, but if you like the smell of strawberry, then go for it! Next you are going to buy some probiotics in capsule or powder form. Those brands of probiotics that come refrigerated are the best, but you can easily use the stuff off the shelf if that's all you can find. Also, choose a product that has multiple strains instead of one strain in it. For this type of application, I don't recommend a liquid probiotic. If you buy the capsule form, make sure that it is the two-part clear capsule that allows you to pull apart the two halves and empty the contents. Enteric probiotics that are sealed pills will not work for this mask because you can't open them.

You can save money on your probiotics by purchasing a high-potency powered form. For example, one serving of a high-

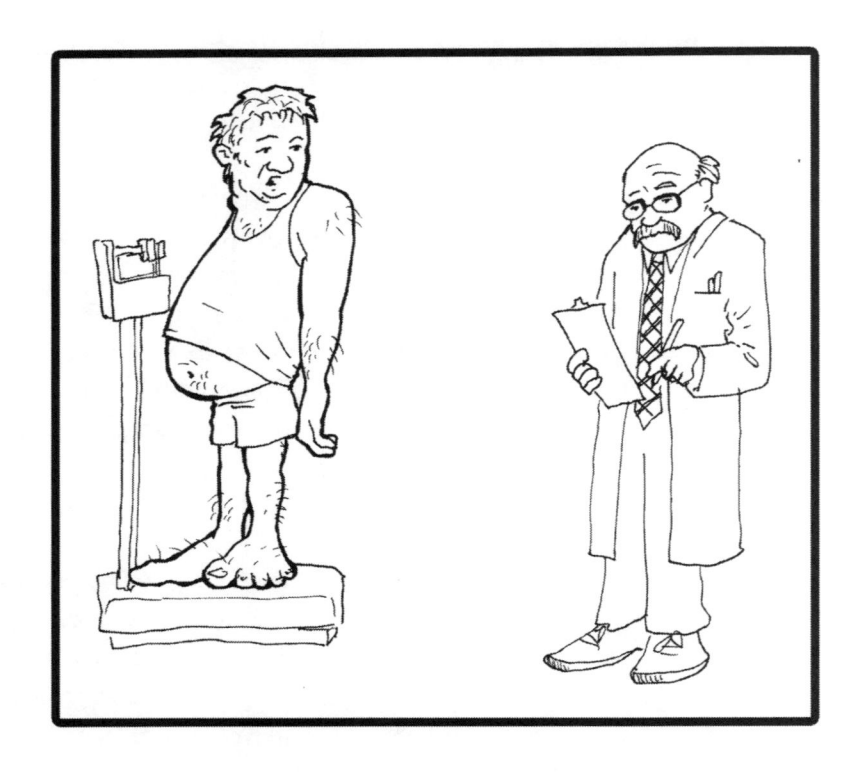

"Doc, I know I've gained a few pounds. But it's all probiotics."
"That's a new one."

potency brand should deliver a couple billion organisms. Most capsule forms usually only contain about a million organisms. Where probiotics are concerned, numbers are king. A million probiotic organisms is such a small amount, it's almost not worth taking as an oral supplement. (Remember, we need a couple of pounds of probiotics in the gut.) It takes about four thousand capsules of the one million serving size to make up one serving of a high-potency probiotic. Once you do the math, you will see that it just isn't cost effective to buy your probiotics at your standard grocery store.

Now, grab a clean bowl and mix a couple billion friendly bacteria into a quarter cup of your yogurt. Stir well to get your medicinal friends well distributed, and apply the mixture to a freshly washed face. Be sure to avoid antibacterial soap for a few days before and after, or it will kill your mask. The next thing you have to do is hang out and indulge yourself in a few of your guilty pleasures while waiting for your yogurt mask to dry. Rinse, and you're done. You should repeat this mask one time weekly for six weeks to gauge the degree of positive impact on your skin from this method.

You may be wondering if this skin care technique is just another bit of magical thinking by the alternative health care world or if it is an approach that is actually going to improve the health of your skin. If you happen to have problem, acne-prone skin, this probiotic mask can really be helpful to you. In fact, there are clinical data to suggest the importance of probiotics in skin health. The idea that topical applications of beneficial bacteria can be an effective treatment for acne has been around since 1912 [315]. There are two main mechanisms by which bacteria on the skin contribute to skin health: (1) as an anti-inflammatory and (2) as a physical barrier. Applying certain types of bacteria to the skin acts like a physical barrier, protecting the skin from invasion by pathogenic bacterial strains. In the field of dermatology, this is called *bacterial interference*. If friendly bacteria are taking up all the open spots in a pore, then there isn't any room for unfriendly bacteria to move in [316]. So, by populating the skin with this probiotic mask, we establish a protective shield over the skin.

Having the right bacteria on the skin also helps to short-circuit the inflammatory response of the skin. Modern research has shown that a strain of stomach acid bacteria commonly found in yogurt (Streptococcus thermophiles) increases ceramide production [317]. Ceramide is a waxy fat that is found in high concentrations in cell membranes. The increase in ceramide was found after applying the lactic acid bacteria to the skin in a cream for seven days. Ceramides are important because they are antimicrobial against propionibacterium acne and have a direct anti-inflammatory effect on the skin. So probiotics are also anti-inflammatory, and this is a good thing for skin.

What follows is yet another reason to consider a probiotic mask as part of good skin hygiene. Topical applications of probiotic bacteria containing *Enterococcus faecalis* for eight weeks reduced inflammatory skin lesions by over 50 percent as compared to a placebo lotion [318]. Just as probiotics are essential for gut health, they also make a huge difference in the health of the skin. You may be wondering why oral supplementation of probiotics isn't enough for skin and why we need topical probiotic applications as well. Keep in mind that the distance between the gut and the skin is huge for a tiny little bacterium. Asking a bacterium that just landed in your stomach to travel to the skin surface is kind of like you walking to Paris. A long way.

The Fruit Shake Mask

One of the common reasons that people seek out the dermatologist is to get a prescription for a topical Retin-A product. These medications are usually available as creams or gels and act as a modulator for skin cell growth and differentiation. Used medically as a treatment for acne, Retin-A-type compounds can be used cosmetically to stimulate skin repair and to reduce the visible signs of aging. However, use of these products can come with some undesirable side effects, including red discoloration, skin flaking, blotchy appearance, and skin thinning. Some of these products also come with birth defect warnings for pregnant women. Because Retin-A derivatives are the same compounds used in many fancy wrinkle creams, many insurance companies may refuse to pay for them (or ask for a letter of medical necessity), even when they are given as a prescription.

Luckily, there is a way that you can get a similar effect at home using all-natural ingredients. A more drastic version of Retin-A treatment is a chemical peel. Medically administered chemical peels work by using strong chemicals to remove the topmost, aged layer of skin. This forces the skin underneath to rejuvenate itself, replacing the missing top layer. This rejuvenation process can result in a reduction of fine lines or certain types of skin discoloration. Instead of using strong chemicals that burn skin or Retin-A products that cause skin thinning, the acids in fruit can be used to slough off the dead skin cells. You can make a mild alpha hydroxy acid skin treatment at home. These types of acids are found in sugarcane, tomato juice, pineapple, and papaya. You can use any combination of these items to make a mild skin treatment that helps to loosen dead skin and reveal younger skin underneath.

To make the fruit shake mask, mix one cup pineapple with one cup papaya in the blender. To test the sensitivity of your skin, apply a small amount to your neck and let it sit for a few minutes. You know how certain fabrics come with a warning to test a small corner with your detergent for color fastness? Your skin is the same way. By applying your mixture to a small area of your skin, you can ensure that your recipe is not too strong. If you have a bad reaction to the fruit acids, then you don't want to apply this treatment to your face. After washing your face, apply this mixture evenly across your face and let it process for two to five minutes. The more sensitive your skin, the less time it takes to get a clinical effect. For a stronger effect, consider adding one to three teaspoons of sugar to your mixture. Sugar contains glycolic acid, which is another member of the alpha

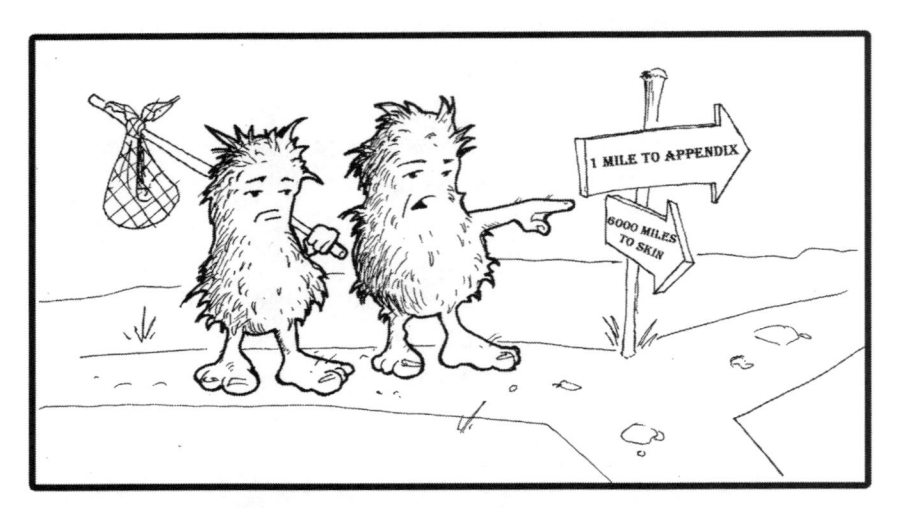

"I hear the weather is nice in the appendix."

hydroxy acid family.

Now you know about the fruit part of the treatment. What about the shake? Now you are going to follow your fruit acid treatment with the miracle mask made from colostrum. The fruit acid treatment helps to break down dead skin cells so that the active ingredients in the colostrum can penetrate more deeply into the layers of the skin.

Afterword

I began this book with a discussion of traditional medical approaches and gave you some reasons why these approaches may not be the best set of methods for curing modern diseases. In addition to the ideas outlined in the introduction, I would like to conclude the book with some final thoughts on this topic. Modern medicine also suffers from another systemic and institutionalized problem: specialization. When you specialize in medicine, you choose a major organ system to be your primary focus for training. Medical students hitting their second year of school are pelted with questions about which specialty they will choose. If future doctors expect to pay back high student loans in a managed care setting, most of them feel forced to choose a higher-paying specialty than the broad focus of family practice.

What does this problem of specialization mean for you directly? As a patient in the end-game system, you have to see different doctors for problems with different organ systems. So, if my heart is beating irregularly, I need to see a cardiologist; if my memory just isn't what it used to be, I have to see a neurologist. But what if a hidden problem is underneath both these organ failures? Lyme disease is an example of a stealth infection that can be the cause of both heart and neurological difficulties. In a best-practice world, the cardiologist and the neurologist would be on the phone together, poring through the medical journals and reviewing clinical interview notes late into the night. But they never do this. And when doctors are trained to investigate only one organ system at a time through specialization, they will miss complex relationships among symptoms. In this example, it is unlikely that the cardiologist or neurologist will consider Lyme disease because they do not generally ask questions about organ systems that are outside their specialty of training.

The solution to the problem of specialization is to now find yourself a good holistic physician. Holistic medicine is a relatively new focus in medical training that encourages the provider to consider the entire body, and relationships among symptoms, all at once. These doctors spend their day looking for underlying causes, combining traditional and alternative therapies, and helping the patient maximize her potential for healing. In this book, I have given you a road map for the journey toward healing, but you also need a guide to tell you what specific path, or combination of therapies, will be right for you. Now that you have taken in the information from this book, your next step is to get an experienced holistic physician playing for your team. There is so much to learn about the field of alternative medicine! New diagnostic tests and clinical studies are being released every day. Get yourself an expert.

Finally, I hope that you will remember that healing is like peeling the layers of an onion. By the time you are motivated to pick up this book, you will have likely developed multiple layers of disease and subclinical infection. Each layer of disease has to be addressed at the rate your body can handle therapy. When you first embark on this healing path, you may even feel like you are moving backward instead of forward because treatment and detox can stir up unexpected physical and emotional symptoms. When things feel dark, I hope you will keep returning to this book for comedic relief, validation, and inspiration. Best of luck in the journey ahead. You can do it.

Acknowledgments

There are so many people to thank whose influence went into this book. Of course, I cannot get to you all. First, I would like to thank all the people who keep me healthy and from whose knowledge I have benefited over the years. Without you and your patient support, this book would never have been written. Special thanks go to all the providers at National Integrated Health Associates in Washington, D.C., and to Dr. Suzette Mikula at Georgetown University Hospital.

Also, I would like to thank my fearless comic artist and loving partner in life, Patrick Geissel. You listened tirelessly to word counts and my latest, greatest ideas for funny pictures. At last, you won't be the only one who gets my jokes.

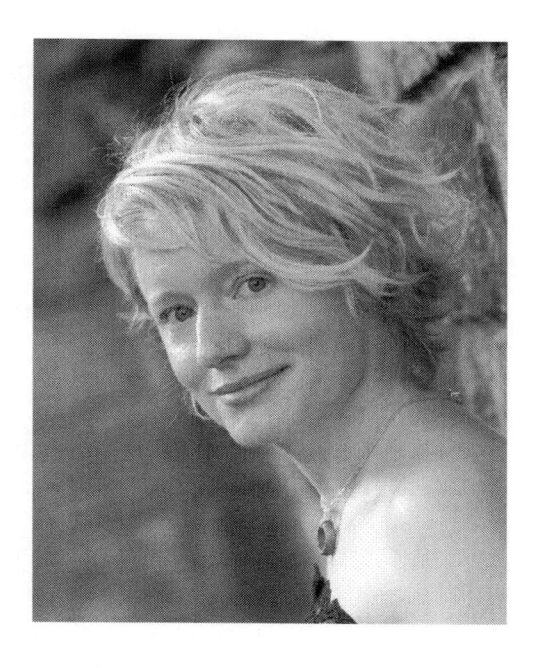

Laura Flynn Geissel, PhD, is a Washington, D.C., based author who holds a master's degree in clinical psychology and a PhD in educational psychology. Geissel spent her career in education, publishing papers in the area of behavioral health while teaching at colleges and universities across the nation. She has now turned her expertise in education to writing books on anti-aging and alternative health. Geissel integrates a solid background in research with her interest in alternative health to produce educational works on the cutting edge of health science. As an author, Geissel explains complex ideas in terms that are easily accessible and often comedic. Geissel's investigations cut through the hype, providing expert opinion on anti-aging, behavioral health, emotional resilience for women, and alternative health models. Geissel's personal research and expert opinions have been published in four scientific journals and *Minority Business Entrepreneur* magazine. She has conducted workshops on mind–body anti-aging strategies, including meditation and holistic wellness. Geissel has also authored a course on Mind-Body Strategies for Stress Reduction that was instituted at a national level. When not writing, the author spends her time painting fine art, enjoying fine dining, and preventing two clever cats from taking over the world.

WORKS CITED

1   Temple NJ. The marketing of dietary supplements in North America: The emperor is (almost) naked. *Journal of Alternative and Complementary Medicine*. 2010;16(7):803-806.

2   Lodén M, Buraczewska I, Halvarsson K. Facial anti-wrinkle cream: Influence of product presentation on effectiveness, a randomized and controlled study. *Skin Research and Technology*. 2007;13(2):189-194.

3   Bodner E. On the origins of ageism among older and younger adults. *International Psychogeriatrics*. 2009;21(6):1003-1014.

4   Hogan MJ, Strasburger VC. Body image, eating disorders, and the media. *Adolescent Medicine: State of the Art Reviews*. 2008;19(3):521-546, x-xi.

5   Gupta MA, Gupta AK, Schork NJ, Voorhees JJ. The aging face: A psychocutaneous perspective. *The Journal of Dermatologic Surgery and Oncology*. 1990;16(10):902-904.

6   Blond A. Impacts of exposure to images of ideal bodies on male body dissatisfaction: A review. *Body Image*. 2008;5(3):244-250.

7   Marshall C, Lengyel C, Utoih A. Body dissatisfaction among middle-aged and older women. *Canadian Journal of Dietetic Practice and Research*. 2012;73(2):e241-e247.

8   Mayes AE, Murray PG, Gunn DA, Tomlin CC, Catt SD, Wen YB, Zhou LP, Wang HQ, Catt M, Granger SP. Environmental and lifestyle factors associated with perceived facial age in Chinese women. *PLos One*. 2010;5(12):e15270.

9   Altabas K, Altabas V, Berković MC, Rotkvić VZ. From cellulite to smooth skin: Is Viagra the new dream cream? *Medical Hypotheses*. 2009;73(1):118-119.

10   Alonso C, Marti M, Martinez V, Rubio L, Parra JL, Coderch L. Antioxidant cosmeto-textiles: Skin assessment. *European Journal of Pharmaceutics and Biopharmaceutics*. 2013;84(1):192-199.

11   Gold MH, Goldman MP, Biron J. Efficacy of novel skin cream containing mixture of human growth factors any cytokines for skin rejuvenation. *Journal of Drugs in Dermatology*. 2007;6(2):197-201.

12   Gold MH, Katz BE, Cohen JL, Biron J. Human growth factor cream and hyaluronic Acid serum in conjunction with micro laser peel: An efficient regimen for skin rejuvenation. *The Journal of Clinical and Aesthetic Dermatology*. 2010;3(12):37-42.

13   Lupo ML, Cohen JL, Rendon MI. Novel eye cream containing a mixture of human growth factors and cytokines for periorbital skin rejuvenation. *Journal of Drugs in Dermatology.* 2007;6(7):775-729.

14   Talbourdet S, Sadick NS, Lazou K, Bonnet-Duquennoy M, Kurfurst R, Neveu M, Heusèle C, André P, Schnebert S, Draelos ZD, Perrier E. Modulation of gene expression as a new skin anti-aging strategy. *Journal of Drugs in Dermatology.* 2007;6(6 Suppl):s25-s33.

15   Nguyen G, Torres A. Systemic antioxidants and skin health. *Journal of Drugs in Dermatology.* 2012;11 (9):e1-4.

16   Cecchi T, Cecchi P, Passamonti P. The first quantitative rating system of the antioxidant capacity of beauty creams via the Briggs-Rauscher reaction: A crucial step towards evidence-based cosmetics. *Analyst.* 2011;136(3):613-618.

17   Mattson MP. Energy intake, meal frequency, and health: A neurobiological perspective. *Annual Review of Nutrition.* 2005;25: 237-260.

18   Marchal J, Perret M, Aujard F. Caloric restriction in primates: How efficient as an anti-aging approach? *Médecine Sciences.* 2012;28(12):1081-1086.

19   Yan L, Gao S, Ho D, Park M, Ge H, Wang C, Tian Y, Lai L, De Lorenzo MS, Vatner DE, Vatner SF. Calorie restriction can reverse, as well as prevent, aging cardiomyopathy. [published online January 20 2013]. *Age.* 2013. http://www.ncbi.nlm.nih.gov/pubmed. Accessed October 5, 2013. PMID:23334601.

20   Parrella E, Maxim T, Maialetti F, Zhang L, Wan J, Wei M, Cohen P, Fontana L, Longo VD. Protein restriction cycles reduce IGF-1 and phosphorylated Ta, and improve behavior performance in an Alzheimer's disease mouse model. *Aging Cell.* 2013;12(2):257-268.

21   Sohal RS, Ku HH, Agarwal S, Forster MJ, Lal H. Oxidative damage, mitochondrial oxidant generation and antioxidant defenses during aging and in response to food restriction in the mouse. *Mechanisms of Ageing and Development.* 1994:74(1-2):121-133.

22   Sohal RS, Agarwal S, Candas M, Forster MJ, Lal H. Effect of age and caloric restriction on DNA oxidative damage in different tissues of C57BL/6 mice. *Mechanisms of Aging and Development.* 1994;76(2-3):215-224.

23   Coleman RJ, Anderson RM, Johnson SC, Kastman EK, Kosmatka KJ, Beasley TM, Allison DB, Cruzen C, Simmons HA, Kemnitz JW, Weindruch R. Caloric restriction delays disease onset and mortality in rhesus monkeys. *Science.* 2009;325(5937):201-204.

24   Mercken EM, Crosby SD, Lamming DW, Jebailey L, Krzysik-Walker S, Villareal D, Capri M, Franceschi C, Zhang Y, Becker K, Sabatini DM, de Cabo R, Fontana L. Calorie restriction in humans inhibits the P13K/AKT pathway and induces a younger transcription profile. [published online April 20 2013]. *Aging cell.* 2013. http://www.ncbi.nlm.nih.gov/pubmed. Accessed August 18, 2013. PMID:23601134.

25   Hinman MR, Ford J, Heyl H. Effects of static magnets on chronic knee pain and physical function: A double-blind study. *Alternative Therapies in Health and Medicine.* 2002;8(4):50-55.

26   Brown CS, Ling FW, Wan JY, Pilla AA. Efficacy of static magnetic field therapy in chronic pelvic pain: A double-blind pilot study. *American Journal of Obstetrics and Gynecology.* 2002;187(6):1581-1587.

27   Wolsko PM, Eisenberg DM, Simon LS, Davis RB, Walleczek J, Mayo-Smith M, Kaptchuk TJ, Phillips RS. Double-blind placebo-controlled trial of static magnets for the treatment of osteoarthritis of the knee: Results of a pilot study. *Alternative Therapies in Health and Medicine.* 2004;10(2):36-43.

28   Eccles NK. A randomized, double-blinded, placebo-controlled pilot study to investigate the effectiveness of a static magnet to relieve dysmenorrhea. *Journal of Alternative and Complementary Medicine.* 2005;11(4):681-687.

29   Weintraub MI, Cole SP. A randomized controlled trial of the effects of a combination of static and dynamic magnetic fields on carpal tunnel syndrome. *Pain Medicine.* 2008;9(5):493-504.

30   Harlow T, Greaves C, White A, Brown L, Hart A, Ernst E. Randomized controlled trial of magnetic bracelets for relieving pain in osteoarthritis of the hip and knee. *BMJ.* 2004;329(7480):1450-1454.

31   Panagos A, Jensen M, Cardenas DD. Treatment of myofascial shoulder pain in the spinal cord injured population using static magnetic fields: A case series. *The Journal of Spinal Cord Medicine.* 2004;27(2):138-142.

32   Khoromi S, Blackman MR, Kingman A, Patsalides A, Matheny LA, Adams S, Pilla AA, Max MB. Low intensity permanent magnets in the treatment of chronic lumber radicular pain. *Journal of Pain and Symptom Management.* 2007;34(4):434-445.

33   Colbert AP, Markov MS, Souder JS. Static magnetic field therapy: Dosimetry considerations. *Journal of Alternative and Complementary Medicine.* 2008; 14(5):577-582.

34   Uruakpa FO, Ismond MA, Akobundu EN. Colostrum and its benefits: A review. *Nutrition Research.* 2002;22(6):755-767.

35   Henderson D. Colostrum is safe and effective for all ages. Center for Nutritional Research. 2005. Unpublished manuscript.

36   Artym J, Zimecki M. The role of lactoferrin in the proper development of newborns. *Postepy Higieny: Medycyny Doswiadczalnej.* 2005;59:421-432.

37   Kelly GS. Bovine colostrums: A review of clinical uses. *Alternative Medicine Review.* 2003;8(4):378-394.

38   Frey R, Odle TG. Colostrum. In: *Gale Encyclopedia of Alternative Medicine.* 2nd ed. Cengage Learning; 2005.

39 Stephan W, Dichtelmüller H, Lissner R. Antibodies from colostrum in oral immunotherapy. *Journal of Clinical Chemistry and Clinical Biochemistry.* 1990;28(1):19-23.

40 Korhonen H, Syvaoja EL, Ahola-Luttila H, Sivela S, Kopola S, Husu J, Kosunen TU. Bactericidal effect of bovine normal and immune serum, colostrum and milk against helicobacter pylori. *The Journal of Applied Bacteriology.* 1995;78(6):655-662.

41 Nord J, Ma P, DiJohn D, Tzipori S, Tacket CO. Treatment with bovine hyperimmune colostrum of cryptosporidial diarrhea in AIDS patients. *AIDS.* 1990;4(6):581-584.

42 Davidson GP, Whyte PB, Daniels E, Franklin K, Nunan H, McCloud PI, Moore AG, More DJ. Passive immunization of children with bovine colostrum containing antibodies to human rotavirus. *Lancet.* 1989;2(8665):709-712.

43 Ciardelli L, Garofoli F, Stronati M, Mazzucchelli I, Avanzini MA, Figar T, Gasparoni A, De Silvestri A, Sabatino G, Chirico G. Human colostrum T lymphocytes and their effector cytokines actively aid the development of the newborn immune system. *International Journal of Immunopathology and Pharmacology.* 2008;21(4):781-786.

44 Struff WG, Sprotte G. Bovine colostrum as a biologic in clinical medicine: A review – part II: Clinical studies. *International Journal of Clinical Pharmacology and Therapeutics.* 2008;46(5):211-225.

45 Park YG, Jeong JK, Moon MH, Lee JH, Lee YJ, Seol JW, Kim SJ, Kang SJ, Park SY. Insulin-like growth factor-1 protects against prion peptide-induced cell death in neuronal cells via inhibition of Bax translocation. *International Journal of Molecular Medicine.* 2012;30(5):1069-1074.

46 Francis GL, Upton FM, Ballard FJ, McNeil KA, Wallace JC. Insulin-like growth factors I and II in bovine colostrum: Sequences and biological activities compared with those of a potent truncated form. *The Biochemcial Journal.* 1988;251(1): 95-103.

47 Skottner A, Arrhenius-Nyberg V, Kanje M, Fryklund L. Anabolic and tissue repair functions of recombinant insulin-like growth factor I. *Acta Paediatrica Scandinavica Supplement.* 1990;367:63-66.

48 Hurley W, Theil PK. Perspectives on immunoglobulins in colostrum and milk. *Nutrients.* 2011;3(4):442-474.

49 Mach JP, Pahud JJ. Secretory IgA, a major immunoglobulin in most bovine external secretions. *Journal of Immunology.* 1971;106:552-563.

50 Moro I, Abo T, Crago SS, Komiyama K, Mestecky J. Natural killer cells in human colostrum. *Cellular Immunology.* 1985;93(2):467-474.

51 Wyatt, D. Anti-aging benefits of Colostrum-LD. Center for Nutritional Research. 2013. Unpublished manuscript.

52   Welch NM. What practicing doctors have to say about colostrum. Center for Nutritional Research Website. http:www.icnr.org. Accessed March 13, 2013.

53   Jensen GS, Patel D, Benson KF. A novel extract from bovine colostrum whey supports innate immune functions. II. Rapid changes in cellular immune function in humans. [published online January 17 2012]. *Preventive Medicine.* 2012. http://www.ncbi.nlm.nih.gov/pubmed. Accessed August 16, 2013. PMID:22285946.

54   Artym J, Zimecki M, Paprocka M, Kruzel ML. Orally administered lactoferrin restores humoral immune response in immunocompromised mice. *Immunology Letters.* 2003;89(1):9-15.

55   Buhmeyer JI. Immune response modulation: Clinically proven immunomodulation and anti-inflammatory spray. Center for Nutritional Research. 2008. Unpublished manuscript.

56   Keech A, Nwabuko U, Chikezie C, Wogu GUE. Peptide immunotherapy: A new treatment direction in HIV/AIDS treatment. Center for Nutritional Research. 2013. Unpublished manuscript.

57   Antonio J, Sanders MS, Van Gammeren D. The effects of bovine colostrum supplementation on body composition and exercise performance in active men and women. *Nutrition.* 2001;17(3):243-247.

58   Institute of Colostrum Research. Sports dietary supplement and colostrum. http://www.colostrumresearch.org. Accessed March 9, 2013.

59   Shing CM, Hunter DC, Stevenson LM. Bovine colostrum supplementation and exercise performance: Potential mechanisms. *Sports Medicine.* 2009;39(12):1033-1054.

60   Buckley J, Abbott M, Martin S, Brinkworth G, Whyte P. Effect of an oral bovine colostrum supplement (intact TM) on running performance. In: *1998 Australian Conference of Science and Medicine October, 1998*; Adelaide, South Australia; 1998.

61   Mero A, Kahkonen J, Nykanen T, Parviainen T, Jokinen I, Takala T, Nikula T, Rasi S, Leppaluoto J. IGF-1, IgA, and IgG responses to bovine colostrum supplementation during training. *Journal of Applied Physiology.* 2002; 93(2):732-739.

62   Vranesic-Bender D. The role of nutraceuticals in anti-aging medicine. *Acta Clinica Croatica.* 2010;49(4):537-544.

63   Ballard FJ, Nield MK, Francis GL, Dahlenburg GW, Wallace JC. The relationship between the insulin content and inhibitory effect of bovine colostrum on protein breakdown in cultured cells. *Journal of Cellular Physiology.* 1982;110(3):249-254.

64   Doillon CJ, Lehance F, Bordeleau LJ, Laplante-Campbell MP, Drouin R. Modulatory effect of a complex fraction derived from colostrum on fibroblast contractibility and consequences on repair tissue. *International Wound Journal.* 2011;8(3):280-290.

65   Kovacs D, Cardinali G, Aspite N, Picardo M. Bovine colostrum promotes growth and migration of the human keratinocyte HaCaT cell line. *Growth Factors*. 2009;27(6):448-455.

66   Bhora FY, Dunkin BJ, Batzri S, Aly HM, Bass BL, Sidawy AN, Harmon JW. Effect of growth factors on cell proliferation and epithelialization in human skin. *Journal of Surgical Research*. 1995;59(2):236-244.

67   Thotathil Z, Jameson MB. Early experience with novel immunomodulators for cancer treatment. *Expert Opinion on Investigational Drugs*. 2007;16(9):1391-1403.

68   Arnold RR, Cole MF, McGhee JR. A bactericidal effect for human lactoferrin. *Science*. 1977;197(4300):263-265.

69   Trumpler U, Straub PW, Rosenmund A. Antibacterial prophylaxis with lactoferrin in neutropenic patients. *European Journal of Clinical Microbiology & Infectious Diseases*. 1989;8(4):310-313.

70   Bullen JJ, Rogers HJ, Griffiths E. Role of iron in bacterial infection. *Current Topics in Microbiology and Immunology*. 1978;80:1-35.

71   Reiter B, Brock JH, Steel ED. Inhibition of Escherichia coli by bovine colostrum and post-colostral milk. II The bacteriostatic effect of lactoferrin on a serum susceptible and serum resistant strain of E. coli. *Immunology*. 1975;28(1):83-95.

72   Zagulski T, Lipinski P, Zagulska A, Broniek S, Jarzabek Z. Lactoferrin can protect mice against a lethal dose of Escherichia coli in experimental infection in vivo. *British Journal of Experimental Pathology*. 1989;70(6):697-704.

73   Ward PP, Piddington CS, Cunningham GA, Zhou X, Wyatt RD, Conneely OM. A system for production of commercial qualities of human lactoferrin: a broad spectrum natural antibiotic. *Biotechnology*. 1995;13(5): 498-503.

74   Berkhout B, Floris R, Recio I, Visser S. The antiviral activity of the milk protein lactoferrin against the human immunodeficiency virus type 1. *Biometals*. 2004;17(3):291-294.

75   Igarashi Y, Skoner DP, Doyle WJ, White MV, Fireman P, Kaliner MA. Analysis of nasal secretions during experimental rhinovirus upper respiratory infections. *The Journal of Allergy and Clinical Immunology*. 1993;92 (5):722-731.

76   Arnold D, Di Biase AM, Marchetti M, Pietrantoni A, Valenti P, Seganti L, Superti F. Antiadenovirus activity of milk proteins: Lactoferrin prevents viral infection. *Antiviral Research*. 2002;53(2):153-158.

77   Drobni P, Naslund J, Evander M. Lactoferrin inhibits human papillomavirus binding and uptake in vitro. *Antiviral Research*. 2004 64(1):63-68.

78   Murphy ME, Kariwa H, Mizutani T, Tanabe H, Yoshimatsu K, Arikawa J, Takashima I. Characterization of in vitro and in vivo antiviral activity of lactoferrin and ribavirin upon hantavirus. *The Journal of Veterinary Medical Science*. 2001;63(6):637-645.

79   Hara K, Ikeda M, Saito S, Matsumoto S, Numata K, Kato N, Tanaka K, Sekihara H. Lactoferrin inhibits hepatitis B virus infection in cultured human hepatocytes. *Hepatology Research.* 2002;24(3):228.

80   Nozaki A, Ikeda M, Naganuma A, Nakamura T, Inudoh M, Tanaka K, Kato N. Identification of a lactoferrin-derived peptide possessing binding activity to hepatitis C virus E2 envelope protein. *Journal of Biological Chemistry.* 2003;278:10162-10173.

81   Green S. Gut mucosa in HIV infection: "Immune milk" Solution. http://www.plosmedicine.org. February 27, 2007. Accessed March 14, 2013.

82   Playford RJ, MacDonald CE, Johnson WJ. Colostrum and milk-derived peptide growth factors for the treatment of gastrointestinal disorders. *American Journal of Clinical Nutrition.* 2000;72(1):5-14.

83   Cartildge SA, Elder JB. Transforming growth factor α and EGF levels in normal human gastrointestinal mucosa. *British Journal of Cancer.* 1989;60(5):657-60.

84   Barnard JA, Beauchamp RD, Russel WE, Dubois RN, Coffey RJ. Epidermal growth factor-related peptides and their relevance to gastrointestinal pathophysiology. *Gastroenterology.* 1995;108(2):564-580.

85   Playford RJ, Floyd DN, MacDonald CE, Calnan DP, Adenekan RO, Johnson W, Goodlad RA, Marchbank T. Bovine colostrum is a health food supplement which prevents NSAID induced gut damage. *Gut.* 1999;44:653-658.

86   Gibbons JA, Kanwar RK, Kanwar JR. Lactoferrin and cancer in different cancer models. *Frontiers in Bioscience (Scholar Edition).* 2011;3:1080-1088.

87   Phillips J, Boiucheix C, Pizza G, Sartorio C, Viza D. Effect of in vitro produced transfer factor on Hodgkin patients. *British Journal of Haematology.* 1978;38(3):430-431.

88   Levin AS, Byers VS, Fudenberg HH, Wybran J, Hackett AJ, Johnston JO, Spitler LE. Osteogenic sarcoma: Immunologic parameters before and during immunotherapy with tumor-specific transfer factor. *The Journal of Clinical Investigation.* 1975;55(3):487-499.

89   Pizza G, De Vinci C, Cuzzocrea D, Menniti D, Aiello E, Maver P, Corrado G, Romagnoli P, Dragoni E, LoConte G, Riolo U, Palareti A, Zucchelli P, Fornarola V, Viza D. A preliminary report on the use of transfer factor for treating stage D3 hormone-unresponsive metastatic prostate cancer. *Biotherapy.* 1996;9(1-3):123-132.

90   Bacsi A, Aguilera-Aguirre L, German P, Kruzel ML, Boldogh I. Colostrinin decreases spontaneous and induced mutation frequencies at the hprt locus in Chinese hamster V79 cells. *Journal of Experimental Therapeutics & Oncology.* 2006;5(4):249-259.

91   Lönnerdal B. Nutritional roles of lactoferrin. *Current Opinion in Clinical Nutrition and Metabolic Care.* 2009;12(3):293-297.

92   Tsuda H, Kozu T, Linuma G, Ohashi Y, Saito D, Saito Y, Akasu T, Alexander DB, Futakuchi M, Fukamachi K, Xu J, Kakizoe T, Ligo M. Cancer prevention by bovine lactoferrin: From animal studies to human trial. *Biometals*. 2010;23(3):399-409.

93   Tuccari G, Barresi G. Lactoferrin in human tumors: Immunohistochemical investigations during more than 25 years. *Biometals*. 2011;24(5):775-784.

94   Goldman AS, Thorpe LW, Goldblum RM, Hanson LA. Anti-inflammatory properties of human milk. *Acta Paediatrica Scandinavica*. 1986;75(5):698-695.

95   Polo J, Campbell JM, Crenshaw J, Rodriguez C, Pujol N, Navarro N, Pujois J. Half-life of porcine antibodies absorbed from a colostrum supplement containing porcine immunoglobulins. *Journal of Animal Science*. 2012;90(Suppl. 4):308-310.

96   All About Colostrum resources page. Center for Nutritional Research Website. http:www.icnr.org. Accessed August 18, 2013.

97   Tangwatcharin P, Khopaibool P. Activity of virgin coconut oil, lauric acid or monolaurin in combination with lactic acid against staphylococcus aureus. *The Southeast Asian Journal of Tropical Medicine and Public Health*. 2012;43(4):969-985.

98   Zhang H, Cui Y, Zhu S, Feng F, Zheng X. Characterization and antimicrobial activity of a pharmaceutical microemulsion. *International Journal of Pharmaceutics*. 2010;395(1-2):154-160.

99   Schlievert PM, Peterson ML. Glycerol monolaurate antibacterial activity in broth and biofilm cultures. [published online July 11 2012]. *PLos One*. 2012. http://www.ncbi.nlm.nih.gov/pubmed. Accessed August 24, 2013. PMID:22808139.

100   Eming SA, Krieg T, Davidson JM. Inflammation in wound repair: molecular and cellular mechanisms. *Journal of Investigative Dermatology*. 2007;127 (3):514-525.

101   De Heredia FP, Gómez-Matinez S, Marcos A. Obesity, inflammation, and the immune system. *The Proceedings of the Nutrition Society*. 2012;71(2):332-338.

102   Purba MB, Kouris-Blazos A, Wattanapenpaiboon N, Lukito W, Rothenberg EM, Steen BC, Wahlqvist ML. Skin wrinkling: Can food make a difference? *Journal of the American College of Nutrition*. 2001;20(1):71-80.

103   Stanford JC, Klein TM, Wolf ED, Allen N. Delivery of substances into cells and tissues using a particle bombardment process. *Particulate Science and Technology: An International Journal*. 1987;5(1):27-37.

104   Walsh G. Therapeutic insulins and their large-scale manufacture. *Applied Microbiology and Biotechnology*. 2005;67(2):151-159.

105   Rahman MA, Ronyai A, Engidaw BZ, Jauncey K, Hwang GL, Smith A, Roderick E, Penman D, Varadi L, Maclean N. Growth and nutritional trials on transgenic Nile tilapia containing an exogenous fish growth hormone gene. *Journal of Fish Biology*. 2001;59 (1):62-78.

106   Cabot RA, Kuhholzer B, Chan AW, Lai L, Park K, Chong K, Schatten G, Murphy CN, Abeydeera LR, Day BN, Prather RS. Transgenic pigs produced using in vitro matured oocytes infected with a retroviral vector. *Animal Biotechnology*. 2001;12(2):205-214.

107   van Dijk SJ, Feskins EJ, Bos MB, Hoelen DW, Heijligenberg R, Bromharr MG, de Groot LC, de Vries JH, Muller M, Afman LA. A saturated fatty acid-rich diet induces and obesity-linked proinflammatory gene expression profile in adipose tissue of subjects at risk of metabolic syndrome. *American Journal of Clinical Nutrition*. 2009;90(6):1656-1664.

108   Murphey DK, Buescher ES. Human colostrum has anti-inflammatory activity in a rat subcutaneous air pouch model of inflammation. *Pediatric Research*. 1993;34(2):208-212.

109   Buescher ES, McWilliams-Koeppen P. Soluble tumor necrosis factor-alpha (TNF-alpha) receptors in human colostrum and milk bind to TNF-alpha and neutralize TNF-alpha bioactivity. *Pediatric Research*. 1998;44(1):37-42.

110   Thompson AB, Bohling T, Payvandi F, Rennard SI. Lower respiratory tract lactoferrin and lysozyme arise primarily in the airways and are elevated in association with chronic bronchitis. *The Journal of Laboratory and Clinical Medicine*. 1990;115(2):148-158.

111   Uchida K, Matsuse R, Tomita S, Sugi K, Saitoh O, Ohshiba S. Immunochemical detection of human lactoferrin in feces as a new marker for inflammatory gastrointestinal disorders and colon cancer. *Clinical Biochemistry*. 1994;27(4):259-264.

112   Lavker R, Kligman A. Chronic heliodermatitis: A morphological evaluation of chronic actinic dermal damage with emphasis on the role of mast cells. *The Journal of Investigative Dermatology*. 1988;90(3):325-330.

113   Conneely OM. Anti-inflammatory activities of lactoferrin. *Journal of the American College of Nutrition*. 2001;20(5):389S-395S.

114   Cumberbatch M, Dearman RJ, Uribe-Luna S, Headon DR, Ward PP, Conneely OM, Kimber I. Regulation of epidermal Langerhans cell migration by lactoferrin. *Immunology*. 2000;100(1):21-8.

115   Kimber I, Cumberbatch M, Dearman RJ, Ward PP, Headon DR, Conneely OM. Regulation by lactoferrin of epidermal Langerhans cell migration. *Advances in Experimental Medicine and Biology*. 1998;443:251-255.

116   Griffiths CE, Cumberbatch M, Tucker SC, Dearman RJ, Andres S, Headon DR, Kimber I. Exogenous topical lactoferrin inhibits allergen-induced Langerhans cell migration and cutaneous inflammation in humans. *The British Journal of Dermatology*. 2001;144(4):715-725.

117   Kanwar JR, Kanwar RK, Sun X, Punj V, Matta H, Morley SM, Parratt A, Puri M, Sehgal R. Molecular and biotechnological advanced in milk proteins in relation to human health. *Current Protein and Peptide Science*. 2009;10(4):308-338.

118 Ward PP, Mendoza-Meneses M, Mulac-Jericevic B, Cunningham GA, Saucedo-Cardenas O, Teng T, Conneely OM. Restricted spatiotemporal expression of lactoferrin during murine embryonic development. *Endocrinology*. 1999;140(4):1852-1860.

119 Ward PP, Mendoza MM, Saucedo-Cardenas O, Teng CT, Conneely OM. Restricted spatiotemporal expression of lactoferrin during murine embryogenesis. *Advances in Experimental Medicine and Biology*. 1998;443: 91-100.

120 Sugi K, Saitoh O, Hirata I, Katsu K. Fecal lactoferrin as a marker for disease activity in inflammatory bowel disease: Comparison with other neutrophil-derived proteins. *The American Journal of Gastroenterology*. 1996;91(5):927-934.

121 Dial EJ, Romero JJ, Headon DR, Lichtenberger LM. Recombinant human lactoferrin is effective in the treatment of Helicobacter felis-infected mice. *The Journal of Pharmacy and Pharmacology*. 2000;52(12):1541-1546.

122 Miyake Y, Sasaki Y, Tanaka K, Ohya Y, Miyamoto S, Matsunaga I, Yoshida T, Hirota Y, Oda H, Osaka Maternal and Child Health Study Group. Fish and fat intake and prevalence of allergic rhinitis in Japanese females: The Osaka Maternal and Child Health Study. *Journal of the American College of Nutrition*. 2007;26(3):279-287.

123 Gil A. Polyunsaturated fatty acids and inflammatory diseases. *Biomedicine and Pharmacotherapy*. 2002;56(8):388-396.

124 Kim HH, Cho S, Lee S, Kim KH, Cho KH, En HC, Chung JH. Photoprotective and anti-skin-aging effects of eicosapentaenoic acid in human skin in vivo. *Journal of Lipid Research*. 2006;47(5):921-930.

125 Jackson MJ, Jackson MJ, McArdle F, Storey A, Jones SA, McArdle A, Rhodes LE. Effects of micronutrient supplements on u.v.-induced skin damage. *The Proceedings of the Nutrition Society*. 2002;61(2):187-189.

126 Pilkington SM, Watson RE, Nicolaou A, Rhodes LE. Omega-3 polyunsaturated fatty acids: Photoprotective macronutrientents. *Experimental Dermatology*. 2011;20(7):537-543.

127 Shingel KL, Faure MP, Azoulay L, Roberge C, Deckelbaum RJ. Solid emulsion gel as a vehicle for delivery of polyunsaturated fatty acids: Implications for tissue repair, demal angiogenesis and wound healing. *Journal of Tissue Engineering and Regenerative Medicine*. 2008;2(7):383-393.

128 Saevik BK, Bergvall K, Holm BR, Saijonmaa-Koulumies LE, Hedhammer A, Larsen S, Kristensen F. A randomized, controlled study to evaluate the steroid sparing effect of essential fatty acid supplementation in the treatment of canine atopic dermatitis. *Veterinary Dermatology*. 2004;15(3):137-145.

129 Rombaldi BJ, de Souza ER, Ferreira CF, Pelufo SP. Fetal and neonatal levels of omega-3: Effects on neurodevelopment, nutrition, and growth. [published online October 17 2012]. *The Scientific World Journal*. 2012. http://www.ncbi.nlm.nih.gov/pubmed. Accessed August 24, 2013. PMID:23125553.

130 Uauy R, Dangour AD. Nutrition in brain development and aging: Role of essential fatty acids. *Nutrition Reviews.* 2006;64(5 Pt 2):S24-S33.

131 Hegarty B, Parker G. Fish oil as a management component for mood disorders – an evolving signal. *Current Opinion in Psychiatry.* 2013;26(1):33-40.

132 Krawczyk K, Rybakowski J. Augmentation of antidepressants with unsaturated fatty acids omega-3 in drug resistant depression. *Psychiatria Polska.* 2012;46(4):585-598.

133 Matsumura K, Noguchi H, Nishi D, Matsuoka Y. The effect of omega-3 fatty acids on psychophysiological assessment for the secondary prevention of posttraumatic stress disorder: An open-label pilot study. *Global Journal of Health Science.* 2011;4(1):3-9.

134 Matsuoka Y, Nishi D, Yonemoto N, Hamazaki K, Matsumura K, Noguchi H, Hashimoto K, Hamazaki T. Tachikawa project for prevention of posttraumatic stress disorder with polyunsaturated fatty acid (TROP): Study protocol for a randomized controlled trial. *BMC Psychiatry.* 2013;13:8.

135 Ribeiro JC, Antunes LM, Aissa AF, Darin JD, De Rosso VV, Mercadante AZ, Bianchi Mde L. Evaluation of the genotoxic and antigenotoxic effects after acute and subacute treatments with açai pulp (Euterpe oleracea Mart.) on mice using the erythrocytes micronucleus test and the comet assay. *Mutation Research.* 2010;695(1-2):22-28.

136 Sabbe S, Verbeke W, Deliza R, Matta VM, Van Damme P. Consumer liking of fruit juices with different açai (Euterpe oleracea Mart.) concentrations. *Journal of Food Science.* 2009;74(5):S171-S176.

137 Guerra JF, Magalhães CL, Costa DC, Silva ME, Pedrosa ML. Dietary açai modulates ROS production by neutrophils and gene expression of liver antioxidant enzymes in rats. [published online June 17 2011]. *Journal of Clinical Biochemistry and Nutrition.* 2011. http://www.ncbi.nlm.nih.gov/pubmed. Accessed August 14, 2013. PMID:22128218.

138 Xie C, Kang J, Li Z, Schauss AG, Badger TM, Nagarajan S, Wu T, Wu X. The açai flavonoid velutin is a potent anti-inflammatory agent: Blockade of LPS-mediated TNF-α and IL-6 production through inhibiting NF-kB activation and MAPK pathway. *The Journal of Nutritional Biochemistry.* 2012;23(9):1184-1191

139 Jensen GS, Ager DM, Redman KA, Mitzner MA, Benson KF, Schauss AG. Pain reduction and improvement in range of motion after daily consumption of an açai (Euterpe oleracea Mart.) pulp-fortified polyphenolic-rich fruit and berry juice blend. [published online April 6 2011]. *Journal of Medicinal Food.* 2011. http://www.ncbi.nlm.nih.gov/pubmed. Accessed August 16, 2013. PMID:21470042.

140 Poulose SM, Fisher DR, Larson J, Bielinski DF, Rimando AM, Carey AN, Schauss AG, Shukitt-Hale B. Anthocyanin-rich açai (Euterpe oleracea Mart.) fruit pulp fractions attenuate inflammatory stress signaling in mouse brain BV-2 microglial cells. *Journal of Agricultural and Food Chemistry.* 2012: 60(4):1084-1093.

141   Moura RS, Ferreira TS, Lopes AA, Pires KM, Nesi RT, Resende AC, Souza PJ, Silva AJ, Borges RM, Porto LC, Valenca SS. Effects of Euterpe oleracea Mart. (açai) extract in acute lung inflammation induced by cigarette smoke in the mouse. *Phytomedicine*. 2012;19(3-4):262-269.

142   Udani JK, Singh BB, Singh VJ, Barrett ML. Effects of açai (Euterpe oleracea Mart.) berry preparation on metabolic parameters in a healthy overweight population: A pilot study. *Nutrition Journal*. 2011;10:45.

143   Sun X, Seeberger J, Alberico T, Wang C, Wheeler CT, Schauss AG, Zou S. Açai palm fruit (Euterpe oleracea Mart.) pulp improves survival of flies on a high fat diet. *Experimental Gerontology*. 2010;45(3):243-251.

144   de Souza MO, Souza E, Silva L, de Brito Magalhães CL, de Figueiredo BB, Costa DC, Silva ME, Pedrosa ML. The hypocholesterolemic activity of açai (Euterpe oleracea Mart.) is mediated by the enhanced expression of the ATP-binding cassette, subfamily G transporters 5 and 8 and low-density lipoprotein receptor genes in the rat. *Nutrition Research*. 2012;32(12):976-984.

145   da Costa CA, de Oliveira PR, de Bem GF, de Cavalho LC, Ognibene DT, da Silva AF, Dos Santos Valença S, Pires KM, da Cunha Sousa PJ, de Moura RS, Resende AC. Euterpe oleracea Mart.-derived polyphenols prevent endothelial dysfunction and vascular structural changes in renovascular hypertensive rats: Role of oxidative stress. *Naunyn-Schmiedeberg's Archives of Pharmacology*. 2012; 385(12):1199-1209.

146   Feio CA, Izar MC, Ihara SS, Kasmas SH, Martins CM, Feio MN, Maués LA, Borges NC, Moreno RA, Póvoa RM, Fonseca FA. Euterpe oleracea (açai) modifies sterol metabolism and attenuates experimentally-induced atherosclerosis. [published online December 3 2011]. *Journal of Atherosclerosis and Thrombosis*. 2011. http://www.ncbi.nlm.nih.gov/pubmed. Accessed August 12, 2013. PMID:22139433.

147   Del Pozo-Insfran D, Percival SS, Talcott ST. Açai (Euterpe oleracea Mart.) polyphenolics in their glycoside and aglycone forms induce apoptosis of HL-60 leukemia cells. *Journal of Agricultural and Food Chemistry*. 2006;54(4):1222-1229.

148   Fragoso MF, Prado MG, Barbosa L, Rocha NS, Barbisan LF. Inhibition of mouse urinary bladder carcinogenesis by açai fruit (Euterpe oleracea Martius) intake. *Plant Foods for Human Nutrition*. 2012;67(3):235-241.

149   Fragoso MF, Romualdo GR, Ribeiro DA, Barbisan LF. Açai (Euterpe oleracea Mart.) feeding attenuates dimethylhydrazine-induced rat colon carcinogenesis. [published online April 15 2013]. *Food and Chemical Toxicology*. 2013. http://www.ncbi.nlm.nih.gov/pubmed. Accessed August 12, 2013. PMID:23597449.

150   Li L, Han AR, Kinghorn AD, Frye RF, Derendorf H, Butterweck V. Pharmacokinetic properties of pure xanthones in comparison to a mangosteen fruit extract in rats. *Planta Medica*. 2013;79(8):646-653.

151   Stern JS, Peerson J, Mishra AT, Sadasiva Rao MV, Rajeswari KP. Efficiency and tolerability of a novel herbal formulation for weight management. *Obesity*. 2013;21(5):921-927.

152   Koh JJ, Qiu S, Zou H, Lakshminarayanan R, Li J, Zhou X, Tang C, Saraswathi P, Verma C, Tan DT, Tan AL, Liu S, Beuerman RW. Rapid bactericidal action of alpha-mangostin against MRSA as an outcome of membrane targeting. [published online September 13 2012]. *Biochimica et Biophysica Acta.* 2013. http://www.ncbi.nlm.nih.gov/pubmed. Accessed August 17, 2013. PMID:22982495.

153   Sudta P, Jiarawapi P, Suksamrarn A, Hongmanee P, Suksamrarn S. Potent activity against multidrug-resistant Mycobacterium tuberculosis of α-mangostin analogs. *Chemical and Pharmaceutical Bulletin.* 2013;61(2):194-203.

154   Jang HY, Kwon OK, Oh SR, Lee HK, Ahn KS, Chin YW. Mangosteen xanthones mitigate ovalbumin-induced airway inflammation in a mouse model of asthma. [published online August 25 2012]. *Food and Chemical Toxicology.* 2012. http://www.ncbi.nlm.nih.gov/pubmed. Accessed August 16, 2013. PMID:22943973.

155   Chomnawang MT, Surassmo S, Nukoolkarn VS, Gritsanapan W. Effect of Garcinia mangostana on inflammation caused by Propionibacterium acnes. *Fitoterapia.* 2007;78(6):401-408.

156   Bumrungpert A, Kalpravidh RW, Chuang CC, Overman A, Martinez K, Kennedy A, McIntosh M. Xanthones from mangosteen inhibit inflammation in human macrophages and in human adipocytes exposed to macrophage-conditioned media. *Journal of Nutrition.* 2010;140(4):842-847.

157   Liu SH, Lee LT, Hu NY, Huange KK, Shih YC, Munekazu I, Li JM, Chou TY, Wang WH, Chen TS. Effects of alpha-mangostin on the expression of anti-inflammatory genes in U937 cells. *Chinese Medicine.* 2012;7(1):19.

158   Udani JK, Singh BB, Barrett ML, Singh VJ. Evaluation of mangosteen juice blend on biomarkers of inflammation in obese subjects: A pilot, dose finding study. *Nutrition Journal.* 2009;8:48.

159   Gutierrez-Orozco F, Chitchumroonchokchai C, Lesinski GB, Suksamrarn S, Failla ML. A-Mangostin: Anti-inflammatory activity and metabolism by human cells. [published online April 11 2013]. *Journal of Agricultural and Food Chemistry.* 2013. http://www.ncbi.nlm.nih.gov/pubmed. Accessed August 14, 2013. PMID:23578285.

160   Márquez-Valadez B, Maldonado PD, Galván-Arzate S, Méndez-Cuesta LA, Pérez-De La Cruz V, Pedraza-Chaverri J, Chánez-Cárdenas ME, Santamaria A. Alpha-mangostin induces changes in glutathione levels associated with glutathione peroxidase activity in rat brain synaptosomes. *Nutritional Neuroscience.* 2012;15(5):13-19.

161   Li G, Thomas S, Johnson JJ. Polyphenols from the mangosteen (Garcinia mangostana) fruit for breast and prostate cancer. *Frontiers in Pharmacology.* 2013;4:80.

162   Kosem N, Ichikawa K, Utsumi H, Moongkarndi P. In vivo toxicity and antitumor activity of mangosteen extract. *Journal of Natural Medicine.* 2013;67(2):255-263.

163   Aisha AF, Abu-Salah KM, Ismail Z, Majid AM. In vitro and in vivo anti-colon cancer effects of Garcinia mangostana xanthones extract. *BMC Complementary and Alternative Medicine*. 2012;12:104.

164   Wang JJ, Sanderson BJ, Zhang W. Significant anti-invasive activities of α-mangostin from the mangosteen pericarp on two human skin cancer cell lines. *Anticancer Research*. 2012;32(9):3805-3816.

165   Liu Z, Antalek M, Nguyen L, Li X, Tian X, Le A, Zi X. The effect of gartanin, a naturally occurring xanthone in mangosteen juice, on the mTOR pathway, autophagy, apoptosis, and the growth of human urinary bladder cancer cell lines. *Nutrition and Cancer*. 2013;65(Suppl. 1):68-77.

166   Johanningsmeier SD, Harris GK. Pomegranate as a functional food and nutraceutical source. *Annual Review of Food Science and Technology*. 2011;2:181-201.

167   Ismail T, Sestili P, Akhtar S. Pomegranate peel and fruit extracts: A review of potential anti-inflammatory and anti-infective effects. [published online July 20 2012]. *Journal of Ethnopharmacology*. 2012. http://www.ncbi.nlm.nih.gov/pubmed. Accessed August 16, 2013. PMID:22820239.

168   Serafini M, Morabito G. The role of polyphenols in the modulation of plasma non-enzymatic antioxidant capacity (NEAC). *International Journal for Vitamin and Nutrition Research*. 2012;82(3):228-232.

169   Shema-Didi L, Sela S, Ore L, Shapiro G, Geron R, Moshe G, Kristal B. One year of pomegranate juice intake decreases oxidative stress, inflammation, and incidence of infections in hemodialysis patients: A randomized placebo-controlled trial. *Free Radical Biology and Medicine*. 2012;53(2):297-304.

170   Espin JC, Larrosa M, Garcia-Conesa MT, Tomás-Barberán F. Biological significance of urolithins, the gut microbial ellagic Acid-derived metabolites: The evidence so far. [published online May 28 2013]. *Evidence-based Complementary and Alternative Medicine*. 2013. http://www.ncbi.nlm.nih.gov/pubmed. Accessed August 12, 2013. PMID:23781257.

171   Ishimoto H, Shibata M, Myojin Y, Ito H, Sugimoto Y, Tai A, Hatano T. In vivo anti-inflammatory and antioxidant properties of ellagitannin metabolite urolithin A. [published online July 29 2011]. *Bioorganic and Medicinal Chemistry Letters*. 2011. http://www.ncbi.nlm.nih.gov/pubmed. Accessed August 16, 2013. PMID:21843938.

172   Balbir-Gurman A, Fuhrman B, Braun-Moscovici Y, Markovitis D, Aviram M. Consumption of pomegranate decreases serum oxidative stress and reduces disease activity in patients with active rheumatoid arthritis: A pilot study. *The Israel Medical Association Journal: IMAJ*. 2011;13(8):474-479.

173   Al-Muammar MN, Khan F. Obesity: The preventive role of the pomegranate (Punica granatum). *Nutrition*. 2012;28(6):595-604.

174 González-Ortiz M, Martinez-Abundis E, Espinel-Bermúdez MC, Pérez-Rubio KG. Effect of pomegranate juice on insulin secretion and sensitivity in patients with obesity. [published online July 28 2011]. *Annals of Nutrition & Metabolism.* 2011. http://www.ncbi.nlm.nih.gov/pubmed. Accessed August 14, 2013. PMID:21811060.

175 Banerjee N, Talcott S, Safe S, Mertens-Talcott SU. Cytotoxicity of pomegranate polyphenolics in breast cancer cells in vitro and vivo: Potential role of miRNA-27a and miRNA-155 in cell survival and inflammation. *Breast Cancer Research and Treatment.* 2012;136(1):21-34.

176 Sreeja S, Santhosh Kumar TR, Lakshmi BS, Sreeja S. Pomegranate extract demonstrate a selective estrogen receptor modulator profile in human tumor cell lines and in vivo models of estrogen deprivation. *The Journal of Nutritional Biochemistry.* 2012;23(7):725-732.

177 Nair V, Dai Z, Khan M, Ciolino HP. Pomegranate extract induces cell cycle arrest and alters cellular phenotype of human pancreatic cancer cells. *Anticancer Research.* 2011;31(9):2699-2704.

178 Wang L, Alcon A, Yuan H, Ho J, Li QJ, Martins-Green M. Cellular and molecular mechanisms of pomegranate juice-induced anti-metastatic effect on prostate cancer cells. *Integrative Biology.* 2011;3(7):742-754.

179 Andersson M, Lindh J. Possible interaction between pomegranate juice and warfarin. *Lakartidningen.* 2012;109(9-10):483.

180 Potterat O. Goji (Lycium barbarum and L. chinense): Phytochemistry, pharmacology and safety in the perspective of traditional uses and recent popularity. *Planta Medica.* 2010;76(1):7-19.

181 Amagase H, Nance DM. A randomized, double-blind, placebo-controlled, clinical study of the general effects of a standardized Lycium barbarum (Goji) juice, GoChi. *Journal of Alternative and Complementary Medicine.* 2008;14(4):403-412.

182 Ren Z, Na L, Xu Y, Rozati M, Wang J, Xu J, Sun C, Vidal K, Wu D, Meydani SN. Dietary supplementation with lacto-wolfberry enhances the immune response and reduces pathogenesis to influenza infection in mice. *The Journal of Nutrition.* 2012;142(8):1596-1602.

183 Wu PS, Wu SJ, Tsai YH, Lin YH, Chao JC. Hot water extracted Lycium barbarum and Rehmannia glutinosa inhibit liver inflammation and fibrosis in rats. *The American Journal of Chinese Medicine.* 2011;39(6):1173-1191.

184 Yu MS, Ho YS, So KF, Yuen WH, Chang RC. Cytoprotective effects of Lycium barbarum against reducing stress on endoplasmic reticulum. *International Journal of Molecular Medicine.* 2006;17(6):1157-1161.

185 Reeve VE, Allanson M, Arun SJ, Domanski D, Painter N. Mice drinking goji berry juice (Lycium barbarum) are protected from UV radiation-induced skin damage via antioxidant pathways. *Photochemical and Photobiological Sciences.* 2010:9(4):601-607.

186   Li XM, Ma YL, Liu XJ. Effects of the Lycium barbarum polysaccharides on age-related oxidative stress in aged mice. *Journal of Ethnopharmacology.* 2007;111(3):504-511.

187   Vidal K, Bucheli P, Gao Q, Moulin J, Shen LS, Wang J, Blum S, Benyacoub J. Immunomodulatory effects of dietary supplementation with a milk-based wolfberry formulation in healthy elderly: A randomized, double-blind, placebo-controlled trial. *Rejuvenation Research.* 2012;15(1):89-97.

188   Vidal K, Benyacoub J, Sanchez-Garcia J, Foata F, Segura-Roggero I, Serrant P, Moser M, Blum S. Intake of a milk-based wolfberry formulation enhances the immune response of young-adult and aged mice. *Rejuvenation Research.* 2010;13(1):47-53.

189   Amagase H, Sun B, Nance DM. Immunomodulatory effects of a standardized Lycium barbarum fruit juice in Chinese older healthy human subjects. *Journal of Medicinal Food.* 2009;12(5):1159-1165.

190   Chen JR, Li EQ, Dai CQ, Yu B, Wu XL, Huang CR, Chen XY. The inducible effect of LBP on maturation of dendritic cells and the related immune signaling pathways in hepatocellular carcinoma (HCC). *Current Drug Delivery.* 2012;9(4):414-420.

191   Luo Q, Li Z, Yan J, Zhu F, Xu RJ, Cai YZ. Lycium barbarum polysaccharides induce apoptosis in human prostate cancer cells and inhibits prostate cancer growth in a xenograft mouse model of human prostate cancer. *Journal of Medicinal Food.* 2009;12(4):695-703.

192   Rivera CA, Ferro CL, Bursua AJ, Gerber BS. Probable interaction between Lycium barbum (Goji) and Warfarin. [published online January 31 2012]. *Pharmacotherapy.* 2012. http://www.ncbi.nlm.nih.gov/pubmed. Accessed August 24, 2013. PMID:22392549.

193   Schöttker B, Haug U, Schomburg L, Köhrle J, Perna L, Müller H, Holleczek B, Brenner H. Strong associations of 25-hydroxyvitamin D concentrations with all-cause, cardiovascular, cancer, and respiratory disease mortality in a large cohort study. *The American Journal of Clinical Nutrition.* 2013;97(4):782-793.

194   Brito A, Cori H, Olivares M, Fernanda Mujica M, Cediel G, López de Romana D. Less than adequate vitamin D status and intake in Latin America and the Caribbean: A problem of unknown magnitude. *Food and Nutrition Bulletin.* 2013;34(1):52-64.

195   Ben-Shoshan M. Vitamin D deficiency/insufficiency and challenges in developing global vitamin D fortification and supplementation policy in adults. *International Journal for Vitamin and Nutrition Research.* 2012;82(4):237-259.

196   Muehleisen B, Gallo RL. Vitamin D in allergic disease: Shedding light on a complex problem. *The Journal of Allergy and Clinical Immunology.* 2013;131(2):324-329.

197 Murr C, Pilz S, Grammer TB, Kleber ME, Meinitzer A, Boehm BO, Marz W, Fuchs D. Vitamin D deficiency parallels inflammation and immune activation, the Ludwigshafen Risk and Cardiovascular Health (LURIC) study. *Clinical Chemistry and Laboratory Medicine.* 2012:50(12):2205-2212.

198 Battersby AJ, Kampmann B, Burl S. Vitamin D in early childhood and the effect on immunity to Mycobacterium tuberculosis [published online July 5 2012]. *Clinical and Developmental Immunology.* 2012. http://www.ncbi.nlm.nih.gov/pubmed. Accessed August 11, 2013. PMID:22829851.

199 Rippel C, South M, Butt WW, Shekerdemian LS. Vitamin D status in critically ill children. *Intensive Care Medicine.* 2012;38(12):2055-2062.

200 Sterling KA, Eftekhari P, Girndt M, Kimmel PL, Raj DS. The immunoregulatory function of vitamin D: Implications in chronic kidney disease. *Nature Reviews: Nephrology.* 2012;8(7):403-412.

201 Field S, Elliott F, Randerson-Moor J, Kukalizch K, Barrett JH, Bishop DT, Newton-Bishop JA. Do Vitamin A derum levels moderate outcome or the protective effect of Vitamin D on outcome from malignant melanoma? [published online April 13 2013]. *Clinical Nutrition.* 2013. http://www.ncbi.nlm.nih.gov/pubmed. Accessed August 12, 2013. PMID:23669635.

202 Walentowicz-Sadlecka M, Sadlecki P, Walentowicz P, Grabiec M. The role of Vitamin D in the carconigenesis of breast and ovarian cancer. *Ginekologia Polska.* 2013;84(4):305-308.

203 Swada M, Carlson JC. Changes in superoxide radical and lipid peroxide formation in the brain, heart, and liver during the lifetime of the rat. *Mechanisms of Aging and Development.* 1987;41(1-2):125-137.

204 Choksi KB, Roberts LJ 2nd, DeFord JH, Rabek JP, Papaconstantinou J. Lower levels of F2-isoprostanes in serum and livers of long-lived Ames dwarf mice. *Biochemical and Biophysical Research Communications.* 2007;364(4):761-764.

205 Rodriguez-Mañas L, El-Assar M, Vallejo S, López-Dóriga P, Solis J, Petidier R, Montes M, Nevado J, Castro M, Góomez-Guerrero C, Peiró C, Sánchez-Ferrer, CF. Endothelial dysfunction in aged humans is related with oxidative stress and vascular inflammation. *Aging Cell.* 2009;8(3):226-238.

206 Dizdaroglu M, Jaruga P. Mechanisms of free radical-induced damage to DNA. *Free Radical Research.* 2012;46(4):382-419.

207 Pageon H, Asselineau D. An in vitro approach to the chronological aging of skin by glycation of the collagen: The biological effect of glycation on the reconstructed skin model. *Annals of the New York Academy of Sciences.* 2005;1043:529-532.

208 Harmon D. A biologic clock: The mitochondria? *Journal of the American Geriatrics Society.* 1972; 20(4):145-147.

209 Davies KJ. Oxidative stress: The paradox of aerobic life. *Biochemical Society Symposium.* 1995;6:1-31.

210 Enomoto A, Endou H. Roles of organic anion transporters (OATs) and a urate transporter (URAT1) in the pathophysiology of human disease. *Clinical and Experimental Nephrology*. 2005;9(3):195-205.

211 Padayatty SJ, Katz A, Wang Y, Eck P, Kwon O, Lee J, Chen S, Corpe C, Dutta A, Levine M. Vitamin C as an antioxidant: Evaluation of its role in disease prevention. *Journal of the American College of Nutrition*. 2003;22(1):18-35.

212 Meister A. Glutathione-ascorbic acid antioxidant system in animals. *The Journal of Biological Chemistry*. 1994;269(13):9397-9400.

213 Herrera E, Barbas C. Vitamin E: Action, metabolism and perspectives. *Journal of Physiology and Biochemistry*. 2001;57 (2):43-56.

214 Tan D, Manchester LC, Reiter RJ, Qi W, Karbownik M, Calvo JR. Significance of melatonin in antioxidative defense system: Reactions and products. *Biological Signals and Receptors*. 2000;9(3-4):137-159.

215 Gruber J, Tang SY, Halliwell B. Evidence for a trade-off between survival and fitness caused by resveratrol treatment of Caenorhabditis elegans. *Annals of the New York Academy of Sciences*. 2007; 1100:530-542.

216 Ferrieres J. The French paradox: Lessons for other countries. *Heart*. 2004;90(1):107-111.

217 Baur JA, Sinclair DA. Therapeutic potential of resveratrol: The in vivo evidence [published online May 26 2006]. *Nature Reviews: Drug Discovery*. 2006;5(6):493-506. http://www.ncbi.nlm.nih.gov/pubmed. Accessed August 11, 2013. PMID:16732220.

218 Del Follo-Martinez A, Banerjee N, Li X, Safe S, Mertens-Talcott S. Resveratrol and quercetin in combination have anticancer activity in colon cancer cells and repress oncogenic microRNA-27a. *Nutrition and Cancer*. 2013;65(3):494-504.

219 Cimino S, Sortino G, Favilla V, Castelli T, Madonia M, Sansalone S, Russo GI, Morgia, G. Polyphenols: Key issues involved in chemoprevention of prostate cancer [published online May 28 2012]. *Oxidative Medicine and Cellular Longevity*. 2012. http://www.ncbi.nlm.nih.gov/pubmed. Accessed August 12, 2013. PMID:22690272.

220 Fang Y, Bradley MJ, Cook KM, Herrick EJ, Nicholl MB. A potential role for resveratrol as a radiation sensitizer for melanoma treatment. [published online March 14 2013]. *Journal of Surgical Research*. 2013. http://www.ncbi.nlm.nih.gov/pubmed. Accessed August 12, 2013. PMID:23522452.

221 Bowers JL, Tyulmenkov VV, Jernigan SC, Klinge CM. Resveratrol acts as a mixed agonist/antagonist for estrogen receptors alpha and beta. *Endocrinology*. 2000;141(10):3657-3667.

222 Walle T, Hsieh F, DeLegge MH, Oatis JE, Walle UK. High absorption but very low bioavailability of oral resveratrol in humans. *Drug Metabolism and Disposition*. 2004;32(12):1377-1382.

223   Athar M, Back JH, Tang X, Kim KH, Kopelovich L, Bickers DR, Kim AL. Resveratrol: A review of preclinical studies for human cancer. *Toxicology and Applied Pharmacology*. 2007;224(3):274-283.

224   Boocock DJ, Faust GE, Patel KR, Schinas AM, Brown VA, Ducharme MP, Booth TD, Crowell JA, Perloff M, Grescher AJ, Steward WP, Brenner DE. Phase I dose escalation pharmacokinetic study in healthy volunteers of resveratrol, a potential cancer chemopreventive agent. *Cancer epidemiology, Biomarkers and Prevention*. 2007;16(6):1246-1252.

225   Szmitko PE, Verma S. Cardiology patient pages: Red wine and your heart. *Circulation*. 2005;111(2):e10-e11.

226   Kopp P. Resveratrol, a phytoestrogen found in red wine: A possible explanation for the conundrum of the "French Paradox? *European Journal of Endocrinology*. 1998;138(6):619-620.

227   Olas B, Wachowicz B. Resveratrol, a phenolic antioxidant with effects on blood platelet functions. *Platelets*. 2005;16(5):251-260.

228   Wang Z, Chen Y, Labinskyy N, Hsieh TC, Ungvari Z, Wu JM. Regulation of proliferation and gene expression in cultured human aortic smooth muscle cells by resveratrol and standardized grape extracts. *Biochemical and Biophysical Research Communications*. 2006;346(1):367-376.

229   Hammargvist F, Luo JL, Cotgreave IA, Anderson K, Wernerman J. Skeletal muscle glutathione is depleted in critically ill patients. *Critical Care Medicine*. 1997;25(1):78-84.

230   Julius M, Lang CA, Gleiberman L, Harburg E, DiFranceisco W, Schork A. Glutathione and morbidity in a community-based sample of elderly. *Journal of Clinical Epidemiology*. 1994;47(9):1021-1026.

231   McPherson RA, Hardy G. Clinical and nutritional benefits of cysteine-enriched protein supplements. *Current Opinion in Clinical Nutrition and Metabolic Care*. 2011;14(6):562-568.

232   Sechi G, Deledda MG, Bua G, Satta WM, Deiana GA, Pes GM, Rosati G. Reduced intravenous glutathione in the treatment of early Parkinson's disease. *Progress in Neuro-psychopharmacology & Biological Psychiatry*. 1996;20(7):1159-1170.

233   Berk M, Copolov D, Dean O, Lu K, Jeavons S, Schapkaitz I, Anderson-Hunt M, Judd F, Katz F, Katz P, Ording-Jespersen S, Little J, Conus P, Cuenod M, Do KQ, Bush AI. N-acetyl cysteine as a glutathione precursor for schizophrenia-a double-blind, randomized, placebo-controlled trial. *Biological Psychiatry*. 2008;64(5):361-368.

234   Van Rammsdonk JM, Hekimi S. Deletion of the mitochondrial superoxide dismutase sod-2 extends lifespan in Caenorhabditis elegans. [published online February 6 2009]. *PLoS Genetics*. 2009. http://www.ncbi.nlm.nih.gov/pubmed. Accessed October 5, 2013. PMID:19197346.

235 Schutz TJ, Zarse K, Voigt A, Urban N, Birringer M, Ristow M. Glucose restriction extends Caenorhabditis elegans life span by inducing mitochondrial respiration and increasing oxidative stress. *Cell Metabolism*. 2007;6(4):280-293.

236 Omenn GS, Goodman GE, Thornquist MD, Balmes J, Cullen MR, Glass A, Keogh JP, Mayskens FL, Valanis B, Williams JH, Barnhart S, Hammer S. Effects of a combination of beta carotene and Vitamin A on lung cancer and cardiovascular disease. *New England Journal of Medicine*. 1996;334(18):1150-1155.

237 Alpha-Tocopherol Beta Carotene Cancer Prevention Study Group. The effect of vitamin E and beta carotene on the incidence of lung cancer and other cancers in male smokers. *New England Journal of Medicine*. 1994;330(15):1029-1035.

238 Miller ER 3rd, Pastor-Barriuso R, Dalal D, Riemersma RA, Appel LJ, Guallar E. Meta-analysis: High dose vitamin E supplementation may increase all-cause mortality. *Annals of Internal Medicine*. 2005;142 (1):37-46.

239 Bjelakovic G, Nikolova D, Simonetti RG, Gluud C. Antioxidant supplements for prevention of gastrointestinal cancers: A systematic review and meta-analysis. *Lancet*. 2004;364(9441):1219-1228.

240 Heart Protection Study Collaborative Group. MRC/BHF Heart Protection Study of antioxidant vitamin supplementation in 20,536 high-risk individuals: A randomized placebo-controlled trial. *Lancet*. 2002;360(9326):23-33.

241 Bjelakovic G, Nagorni A, Nikolova D, Simonetti RG, Bjelakovic M, Gluud C. Meta-analysis: Antioxidant supplements for primary and secondary prevention of colorectal adenoma. *Ailment Pharmacological Therapy*. 2006;24:281-291.

242 Age-Related Eye Disease Study Research Group. A randomized, placebo-controlled, clinical trial of high-dose supplementation with vitamins C and E and beta carotene for age-related cataract and vision loss: AREDS report no. 9. *Archives of Ophthalmology*. 2001; 119(10):1439-1452.

243 Hemilä H, Chalker E. Vitamin C for preventing and treating the common cold. *Cochrane Database of Systemic Reviews*. 2013;1:CD000980.

244 Bjelakovic G, Nikolova D, Gluud LL, Simonetti RG, Gluud C. Mortality in randomized trials of antioxidant supplements for primary and secondary prevention: Systemic review and meta-analysis. *Journal of the American Medical Association*. 2007;297(8):842-857.

245 Ristow M, Schmeisser S. Extending life span by increasing oxidative stress. *Free Radical Biology and Medicine*. 2011;51(2):327-336.

246 Pugliese PT. The Skin's Antioxidant Systems. *Dermatology Nursing*. 1988;10(6):401-416.

247 McGilvray ID, Rotstein OD. Antioxidant modulation of skin inflammation: Preventing inflammatory progression by inhibiting neutrophil influx. *Canadian Journal of Surgery*. 1999;42(2):109.

248   Sood S, Arora B, Bansal S, Muthuramen A, Gill N, Arora R, Bali M, Sharma P. Antioxidant, anti-inflammatory and analgesic potential of the Citrus decumana L. peel extract. *Inflammopharmacology.* 2009;17(5):267-274.

249   Koedrith P, Kim H, Weon JI, Seo YR. Toxicogenomic approaches for understanding molecular mechanisms of heavy metal mutagenicity and carcinogenicity. [published online March 13 2013]. *International Journal of Hygiene and Environmental Health.* 2013. http://www.ncbi.nlm.nih.gov/pubmed. Accessed August 17, 2013. PMID:23540489.

250   Huang HH, Huang JY, Lung CC, Wu CL, Ho CC, Sun YH, Ko PC, Su SY, Chen SC, Liaw YP. Cell-type specificity of lung cancer associated with low-dose soil heavy metal contamination in Taiwan: An ecological study. *BMC Public Health.* 2013;13:330.

251   Nikolaidis C, Orfanidis M, Hauri D, Mylonas S, Constantinidis T. Public health risk assessment associated with heavy metal and arsenic exposure near an abandoned mine. [published online February 19 2013]. *International Journal of Environmental Health Research.* 2013. http://www.ncbi.nlm.nih.gov/pubmed. Accessed August 18, 2013. PMID:23418882.

252   Fakour H, Esmaili-Sari A, Zayeri F. Mercury exposure assessment in Iranian women's hair of a port town with respect to fish consumption and amalgam fillings. *The Science of the Total Environment.* 2010;408(7):1538-1543.

253   Kruzikova K, Kensova R, Blahova J, Harustiakova D, Svobodova Z. Using human hair as an indicator for exposure to mercury. *Neuro Endocrinology Letters.* 2009;30(Suppl 1):177-181.

254   Khlifi R, Olmedo P, Gil F, Hammami B, Chakroun A, Rebai A, Hamza-Chaffai A. Arsenic, cadmium, chromium, and nickel in cancerous and healthy tissues from patients with head and neck cancer. [published online March 15 2013]. *The Science of the Total Environment.* 2013. http://www.ncbi.nlm.nih.gov/pubmed. Accessed August 16, 2013. PMID:23500399.

255   Geier DA, Carmody T, Kern JK, King PG, Geier MR. A significant relationship between mercury exposure from dental amalgams and urinary porphyrins: A further assessment of the Casa Pia Children's Dental Amalgam Trial. [published online November 5 2010]. *Biometals.* 2011. http://www.ncbi.nlm.nih.gov/pubmed. Accessed August 14, 2013. PMID:21053054.

256   Muran PJ. Mercury elimination with oral DMPS, DMSA, vitamin C, and glutathione: An observational clinical review. *Alternative Therapies in Health and Medicine.* 2006;12(3):70-75.

257   Liu XL, Wang HB, Sun CW, Xiong XS, Chen Z, Li ZS, Han B, Yang G. The clinical analysis of mercury poisoning in 92 cases. *Zhonghua Nei Ke Za Zhi.* 2011;50(8):687-689.

258   Shargorodsky J, Curhan SG, Henderson E, Eavey R, Curhan GC. Heavy metals exposure and hearing loss in US adolescents. *Archives of Otolaryngology Head Neck Surgery.* 2011;137(12):1183-1189.

259 Desoto MC, Hitlan RT. Sorting out the spinning of autism: Heavy metals and the question of incidence. *Acta Neurobiologiae Experimentalis.* 2010;70(2):165-176.

260 Flora SJ, Mittal M, Mehta A. Heavy metal induced oxidative stress & its possible reversal by chelation therapy. *Indian Journal of Medical Research.* 2008;128(4):501-523.

261 Mutter J. Is dental amalgam safe for humans? The opinion of the scientific committee of the European Commission. *Journal of Occupational Medicine and Toxicology.* 2011;6(1):2.

262 Geier DA, Carmody T, Kern JK, King PG, Geier MR. A significant dose-dependent relationship between mercury exposure from dental amalgams and kidney integrity biomarkers: A further assessment of the Casa Pia Children's Dental Amalgam Trial. [published online August 14 2012]. *Human and Experimental Toxicology.* 2013. http://www.ncbi.nlm.nih.gov/pubmed. Accessed August 14, 2013. PMID:22893351.

263 Richardson GM, Wilson R, Allard D, Purtill C, Douma S, Gravière J. Mercury exposure and risks from dental amalgam in the US population. *The Science of the Total Environment.* 2011;409(20):4257-4268.

264 Geier DA, Carmody T, Kern JK, King PG, Geier MR. A dose-dependent relationship between mercury exposure from dental amalgams and urinary mercury levels: A further assessment Casa Pia Children's Dental Amalgam Trial. [published online July 29 2011]. *Human and Experimental Toxicology.* 2012. http://www.ncbi.nlm.nih.gov/pubmed. Accessed August 14, 2013. PMID:21803780.

265 Norouzi E, Bahramifar N, Ghasempouri SM. Effect of teeth amalgam on mercury levels in the colostrums human milk in Lenjan. *Environmental Monitoring and Assessment.* 2012;184(1):375-380.

266 Rai UN, Singh NK, Upadhyay AK, Verma S. Chromate tolerance and accumulation in chlorella vulgaris L: Role of antioxidant enzymes and biochemical changes in detoxification of metals. *Bioresource Technology.* 2013;136:604-609.

267 Rao PH, Kumar RR, Raghaven BG, Subramanian VV, Sivasubramanian V. Is phycovolatilization of heavy metals a probable (or possible) physiological phenomenon? An in situ pilot-scale study at a leather-processing chemical industry. *Water Environment Research.* 2011;83(4):291-297.

268 Queiroz ML, da Rocha MC, Torello CO, de Souza Queiroz J, Bincoletto C, Morgano MA, Romano MR, Paredes-Gamero EJ, Barbosa CM, Calgarotto AK. Chlorella vulgaris restores bone marrow cellularity and cytokine production in lead-exposed mice. *Food and Chemical Toxicology.* 2011;49(11):2934-2941.

269 Uchikawa T, Ueno T, Hasegawa T, Maruyama I, Kumamoto S, Ando Y. Parachlorella beyerinckii accelerates lead excretion in mice. *Toxicology and Industrial Health.* 2009;25(8):551-556.

270   Uchikawa T, Kumamoto Y, Maruyama I, Kumamoto S, Ando Y, Yasutake A. Enhanced elimination of tissue methylmercury in Parachlorella beijerinckii-fed mice. *The Journal of Toxicological Sciences*. 2011;36(1):121-126.

271   Chisolm JJ, Jr. Safety and efficacy of meso-2,3-dimercaptosuccinic acid (DMSA) in children with elevated blood lead concentrations. *Journal of Toxicology, Clinical Toxicology*. 2000;38(4):365-375.

272   Bridges CC, Joshee L, Zalups RK. Effect of DMPS and DMSA on the placental and fetal disposition of methylmercury. *Placenta*. 2009;30(9):800-805.

273   Vamnes JS, Eide R, Isrenn R, Hől PJ, Gjerdet NR. Diagnostic value of a chelating agent in patients with symptoms allegedly caused by amalgam fillings. *Journal of Dental Research*. 2000;79(3):868-874.

274   Kidd RF. Results of dental amalgam removal and mercury detoxification using DMPS and neural therapy. *Alternative Therapies in Health and Medicine*. 2000;6(4):49-55.

275   Winker R, Schaffer AW, Konnaris C, Barth A, Giovanoli P, Osterode W, Rüdiger HW, Wolf C. Health consequences of an intravenous injection of metallic mercury. *International Archives of Occupational and Environmental Health*. 2002;75(8):581-586.

276   Brandão R, Santos FW, Farina M, Zeni G, Bohrer D, Rocha JB, Nogueira CW. Antioxidants and metallothionein levels in mercury-treated mice. *Cell Biology and Toxicology*. 2006;22(6):429-438.

277   Odenwald MA, Turner JR. Intestinal permeability defects: Is it time to treat? [published online July 12 2013]. *Clinical gastroenterology and hepatology*. 2013. http://www.ncbi.nlm.nih.gov/pubmed. Accessed August 14, 2013. PMID:23851019.

278   Rapin JR, Wiernsperger N. Possible links between intestinal permeability and food processing: A potential therapeutic niche for glutamine. *Clinics*. 2010;65(6):635-643.

279   Barbara G, Zecchi L, Barbaro R, Cremon C, Bellacosa L, Marcellini M, De Giorgio R, Corinaldesi R, Stanghellini V. Mucosal permeability and immune activation as potential therapeutic targets of probiotics in irritable bowel syndrome. *Journal of Clinical Gastroenterology*. 2012;46(Suppl):S52-S55.

280   Gecse K, Róka R, Séra T, Rosztóczy A, Annaházi A, Izbéki F, Nagy F, Molnár T, Szepes Z, Pávics L, Bueno L, Wittmann T. Leaky gut in patients with diarrhea-predominant irritable bowel syndrome and inactive ulcerative colitis. [published online December 14 2011]. *Digestion*. 2012. http://www.ncbi.nlm.nih.gov/pubmed. Accessed August 14, 2013. PMID:22179430.

281   Maes M, Coucke F, Leunis JC. Normalization of the increased translocation of endotoxin from gram negative enterobacteria (leaky gut) is accompanied by a remission of chronic fatigue syndrome. *Neuro Endocrinology Letters*. 2007;28(6):739-744.

282   Brenchley JM, Price DA, Schacker TW, Asher TE, Silvestri G, Rao S, Kazzaz Z, Bornstein E, Lambotte O, Altmann D, Blazar BR, Rodriquez B, Teixeira-Johnson L, Landay A, Martin JN, Hecht FM, Picker LJ, Lederman MM, Deeks SG, Douek DC. Microbial translocation is a cause of systemic immune activation in chronic HIV infection. *Nature Medicine.* 2006;12(12):1365-1371.

283   Plettenberg A, Stoehr A, Stellbrink HJ, Albrecht H, Meigel W. A preparation from bovine colostrum in the treatment of HIV-positive patients with chronic diarrhea. *The Clinical Investigator.* 1993;71(1)42-45.

284   Chapman TM, Plosker GL, Figgitt DP. Spotlight on VSL #3 probiotic mixture in chronic inflammatory bowel diseases. *Biodrugs.* 2007;21(1):61-63.

285   Tursi A, Brandimarte G, Papa A, Giglio A, Elisel W, Giorgetti GM, Forti G, Morini S, Hassan C, Pistoia MA, Modeo ME, Rodino' S, D'Amico T, Sebkova L, Sacca' N, Di Giulio E, Luzza F, Imeneo M, Larussa T, Di Rosa S, Annese V, Danese S, Gasbarrini A. Treatment of relapsing mild-to-moderate ulcerative colitis with the probiotic VSL #3 as adjunctive to a standard pharmaceutical treatment: A double-blind, randomized, placebo-controlled study. *The American Journal of Gastroenterology.* 2010;105(10):2218-2227.

286   Sood A, Midha V, Makharia GK, Ahuja V, Singal D, Goswami P, Tandon RK. The probiotic preparation, VSL #3 induces remission in patients with mild-to-moderately active ulcerative colitis. *Clinical Gastroenterology and Hepatology.* 2009;7(11):1202-1209.

287   Selinger CP, Bell A, Cairns A, Lockett M, Sebastian S, Haslam N. Probiotic VSL#3 prevents antibiotic-associated diarrhea in a double-blind randomized, placebo-controlled trial. *The Journal of Hospital Infection.* 2013;84(2):159-165.

288   Bowen JM, Stringer AM, Gibson RJ, Yeoh AS, Hannam S, Keefe DM. VSL #3 probiotic treatment reduces chemotherapy-induced diarrhea and weight loss. *Cancer, Biology, and Therapy.* 2007;6(9):1449-1454.

289   Dharmani P, De Simone C, Chadee K. The probiotic mixture VSL #3 accelerates gastric ulcer healing by stimulating vascular endothelial growth factor. [published online March 6 2013]. *PLoS One.* 2013. http://www.ncbi. nlm.nih.gov/pubmed. Accessed August 12, 2013. PMID:23484048.

290   Kuo CH, Lee SH, Chen KM, Lii CK, Liu CY. Effect of garlic oil on neutrophil infiltration in the small intestine of endotoxin-injected rats and its association with levels of soluble and cellular adhesion molecules. *Journal of Agricultural and Food Chemistry.* 2011;59(14):7717-7725.

291   Tessema B, Mulu A, Kassu A, Yismaw G. An in vitro assessment of the antibacterial effect of garlic (Allium sativum) on bacterial isolates from wound infections. *Ethiopian Medical Journal.* 2006;44(4):385-389.

292   Goncagul G, Ayaz E. Antimicrobial effect of garlic (Allium sativum). *Recent Patents on Anti-infective Drug Discovery.* 2010;5(1):91-93.

293   Reid K, Toben C, Fakler P. Effect of garlic on serum lipids: An updated meta-analysis. *Nutrition Reviews.* 2013;71(5):282-299.

294   Filocamo A, Nueno-Palop C, Bisignano C, Mandalari G, Narbad A. Effect of garlic powder on the growth of commensal bacteria from the gastrointestinal tract. [published online June 15 2012]. *Phytomedicine*. 2012. http://www.ncbi.nlm.nih.gov/pubmed. Accessed August 12, 2013. PMID:22480662.

295   O'Gara EA, Maslin DJ, Nevill AM, Hill DJ. The effect of simulated gastric environments on the anti-Helicobacter activity of garlic oil. *Journal of Applied Microbiology*. 2008;104(5):1324-1331.

296   Lu X, Rasco BA, Jabal JM, Aston DE, Lin M, Konkel ME. Investigating antibacterial effects of garlic (Allium sativum) concentrate and garlic-derived organosulfur compounds on Campylobacter jejuni by using Fourier transform infrared spectroscopy, Raman spectroscopy, and electron microscopy. *Applied and Environmental Microbiology*. 2011;77(15):5257-5269.

297   Tedeschi P, Maietti A, Boggian M, Vecchiati G, Brandolini V. Fungitoxicity of lyophilized and spray-dried garlic extracts. *Journal of Environmental Science and Health: Part B*. 2007;42(7):795-799.

298   Luo DQ, Guo JH, Wang FJ, Jin ZX, Cheng XL, Zhu JC, Peng CQ, Zhang C. Anti-fungal efficacy of polybutylcyanoacrylate nanoparticles of allicin and comparison with pure allicin. *Journal of Biomaterial Science*. 2009;20(1):21-31.

299   Ogita A, Nagao Y, Fujita K, Tanaka T. Amplification of vacole-targeting fungicidal activity of antibacterial antibiotic polymyxin B by allicin, an allyl sulfur compound from garlic. *The Journal of Antibiotics*. 2007;60(8):511-518.

300   Süntar IP, Akkol EK, Baykal T. Assessment of anti-inflammatory and antinociceptive activities of Olea europaea L. *Journal of Medicinal Food*. 2010;13(2):352-356.

301   Amin A, Khan MA, Shah S, Ahmad M, Zafar M, Hameed A. Inhibitory effects of Olea ferruginea crude leaves extract against some bacterial and fungal pathogen. *Pakistan Journal of Pharmaceutical Science*. 2013;26(2):251-254.

302   Pereira AP, Ferreira IC, Marcelino F, Valentão P, Andrade PB, Seabra R, Estevinho L, Bento A, Pereira JA. Phenolic compounds and antimicrobial activity of olive (Olea europaea L. Cv. Cobrançosa) leaves. *Molecules*. 2007;12(5):1153-1162.

303   Sudjana AN, D'Orazio C, Ryan V, Rasool N, Ng J, Islam N, Riley TV, Hammer KA. Antimicrobial activity of commercial Olea europaea (olive) leaf extract. *International Journal of Antimicrobial Agents*. 2009;33(5):461-463.

304   Markin D, Duek L, Berdicevsky I. In vitro antimicrobial activity of olive leaves. *Mycoses*. 2003;46(3-4):132- 136.

305   Friedman M, Henika PR, Levin CE. Bactericidal activities of health-promoting, food-derived powders against the foodborne pathogens Escherichia coli, Listeria monocytogenes, Salmonella enterica, and Staphylococcus aureus. *Journal of Food Science*. 2013;78(2):M270-M275.

306   Oikarinen A. Aging of the skin connective tissue: how to measure the biochemical and mechanical properties of aging dermis. *Photodermatology, Photoimmunology and Photomedicine*. 1994;10(2):47-52.

307 Moschella S, Hurley H. Aging and Its Effects on the Skin. In: *Dermatology: Third Edition.* Philadelphia: W.B. Saunders Company;2002.

308 Ekiz O, Yüce G, Ulaşli SS, Ekiz F, Yüce S, Başar O. Factors influencing skin aging in a Mediterranean population from Turkey. *Clinical and Experimental Dermatology.* 2012;37(5):492-496.

309 Yasui T, Yonetsu M, Tanaka R, Tanaka Y, Fukushima S, Yamashita T, Ogura Y, Hirao T, Murota H, Araki T. In vivo observation of age-related structural changes of dermal collagen in human facial skin using collagen-sensitive second harmonic generation microscope equipped with 1250-nm mode-locked Cr: Forsterite laser. *Journal of Biomedical Optics.* 2013;18(3):31108.

310 Fisher GJ. The Pathophysiology of Photoaging of the Skin. *Cutis.* 2005;75(2 Supplement):5-9.

311 Demierrr MF, Brooks D, Koh HK, Geller AC. Public knowledge, awareness, and perceptions of the association between skin aging and smoking. *Journal of the American Academy of Dermatology.* 1999;41(1):27-30.

312 Koh JS, Kang H, Choi SW, Kim HO. Cigarette smoking associated with premature facial wrinkling: image analysis of facial skin replicas. *International Journal of Dermatology.* 2002;41(1):21-27.

313 Seité S, Fourtanier AM. The benefit of daily photoprotection. *Journal of the American Academy of Dermatology.* 2008;58(5 Supplement 2):S160-S166.

314 Devos SA, Van der Endt JD, Broeckx W, Vandaele M, del Marmol V, Roseeuw D, Maselis T. Sunscreen use and skin protection behavior on the Belgian beach: A comparison 9 years later. *European Journal of Cancer Prevention.* 2012;21(5):474-477.

315 Peyri J. Topical bacteriotherapy of the skin. *Journal of Cutaneous Disease.* 1912;30:688-689.

316 Brook I. Bacterial interference. *Critical Reviews in Microbiology.* 1999;25(3):155-172.

317 Pavicic T, Wollenweber U, Farwick M, Korting HC. Anti-microbial and anti-inflammatory activity and efficacy of phytosphingosine: an in vitro an in vivo study addressing acne vulgaris. *International Journal of Cosmetic Science.* 2007;29(3):181-190.

318 Kang BS, Seo JG, Lee GS, Kim JH, Kim SY, Han YW, Kang H, Kim HO, Rhee JH, Chung MJ, Park YM. Antimicrobial activity of enterocins from Enterococcus faecalis SL-5 against propionibacterium acnes, the causative agent in acne vulgaris, and its therapeutic effect. *Journal of Microbiology.* 2009;47(1):101-109.

GET CONNECTED
www.facebook.com/LauraGeisselReads

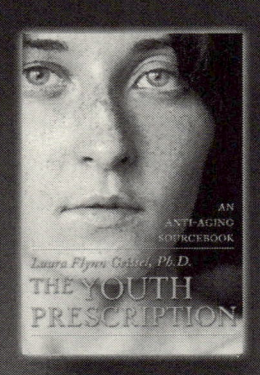

Join a like-minded community of people
who care about natural ways of healing
AND
Get the latest posts from Dr. Geissel
on antiaging science.

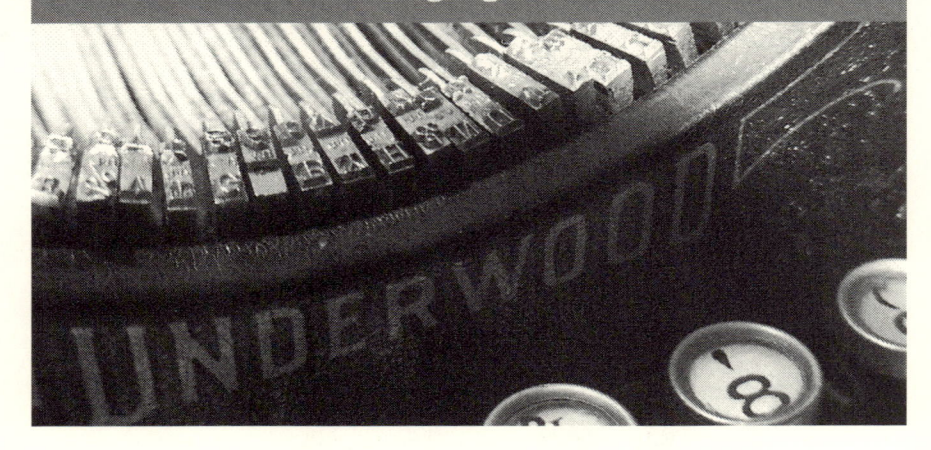

WANT MORE BY LAURA GEISSEL?

www.LauraGeisselReads.com

Made in the USA
Charleston, SC
21 April 2014